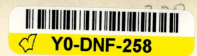

TOTAL BODY GUIDE

Thank you for purchasing Women's Health Total Body Guide. We are very interested in finding out a little more about you so we can tailor future publications to your needs and interests. When you're finished, just tear out the survey, and mail it by October 31, 2003.

Mail to: PREVENTION'S TOTAL BODY GUIDE/Reader Survey
Attn: Mary Banyas, 33 E. Minor St., Emmaus, PA 18098

Thanks—we look forward to hearing from you!

WHAT DID YOU THINK?

1. Overall, how would you rate this publication: *Total Body Guide?*
(Please circle your response.)
1 = Excellent
2 = Very good
3 = Good
4 = Fair
5 = Poor

2. Which of the following did you do prior to actually purchasing this publication?
(Please check all that apply.)
❏ Looked at the cover
❏ Examined the table of contents
❏ Skimmed several of the chapters
❏ Flipped through the whole publication
❏ Checked the price
❏ Compared it to other publications

3. Which of the following cover lines made you want to buy this issue of *Total Body Guide?*
(Please check up to three choices.)
❏ FAB ABS
  Results in 4 weeks
❏ TURN UP THE BURN
  10-minute fast results workout
❏ LOSE ALL THE WEIGHT
  A low-carb plan you'll love
❏ CELLULITE BLITZ
  What really works

4. Please rate each of the following sections in this publication.
(Use the scale to choose the number that best represents your opinion, then write the number on the line.)
1 = Liked it very much
2 = Liked it somewhat
3 = Disliked it somewhat
4 = Did not like it at all
5 = Didn't read it

____ Part 1: Get firm fast! p. 2
____ Part 2: Cardio blast! p. 38
____ Part 3: Stretch it out! p. 64
____ Part 4: Eat to lose! p. 84
____ Part 5: Real meals you'll love p. 108
____ Part 6: Keep the drive alive! p. 154
____ Part 7: Bonus beauty section! p. 168

5. How would you rate the price you paid for this publication?
(Please check one box.)
❏ Too high for the amount of information it contains
❏ Just right for the amount of information it contains
❏ Too low for the amount of information it contains

YOUR READING INTERESTS

6. Which of the following magazines do you subscribe to or typically buy at the store?
(Please circle the number for your response to each magazine.)

	SUBSCRIBE	BUY
Glamour	1	2
Good Housekeeping	1	2
Health	1	2
Ladies' Home Journal	1	2
More	1	2
Prevention	1	2
Reader's Digest	1	2
Redbook	1	2
Self	1	2
Shape	1	2

continued on next page

7. After reading this publication, how likely are you to subscribe to *Prevention* magazine?
(Please circle your response.)
1 = Very likely
2 = Somewhat likely
3 = Not very likely
4 = Not at all likely
5 = I already subscribe

8. Which of these *Prevention* publications would interest you?
(Please check up to three choices.)
❑ Doctor's Book of Home Remedies
❑ Eat Up/Slim Down Cookbook
❑ Healing with Vitamins
❑ Medical Breakthroughs
❑ Natural Healing Guide
❑ Nature's Drugstore
❑ Nutrition News
❑ Outwit Your Weight
❑ Stress-Free Living
❑ *Prevention*'s Ultimate Nutrition Guide
❑ Women's Health Today
❑ Yoga
❑ Your 30-Day Weight Loss Planner

9. Which of these condition-specific publications would interest you?
(Please check up to three choices.)
❑ Outsmart Allergies
❑ Outsmart Asthma
❑ Outsmart Arthritis
❑ Outsmart Cancer
❑ Outsmart Cholesterol

❑ Outsmart Disease: Complete A-to-Z Guide
❑ Outsmart Depression
❑ Outsmart Heart Disease
❑ Outsmart Your Hormones
❑ Outsmart Infertility
❑ Outsmart Menopause
❑ Outsmart Osteoporosis
❑ Outsmart Pain

10. What common ailments are you most interested in learning more about? *(Please check up to three choices.)*
❑ Back pain
❑ Foot care
❑ Heartburn
❑ Headache
❑ Vision
❑ Other _____

11. Have you purchased any of these *Prevention Guides* in the past year?
❑ Outsmart Arthritis
❑ Outsmart Diabetes
❑ Outsmart Diabetes Cookbook
❑ Outsmart Heart Disease
❑ Outsmart Heart Disease Cookbook
❑ Low-Carb Weight Loss
❑ 30-Day Weight Loss Planner
❑ Fit and Firm
❑ Walking Fit
❑ Weight Loss

ABOUT YOU
12. ❑ Male   ❑ Female

13. What is your age? _____

14. How much weight would you like to lose?
(Please circle your response.)
1 = None, I'm at my ideal weight
2 = 5–10 lb
3 = 10–25 lb
4 = 25–50 lb
5 = 50+ lb

15. What is your education?
(Please circle your response.)
1 = High school graduate (or less)
2 = Some college/associate degree
3 = College degree (or more)

16. Household income before taxes:
(Please circle your response.)
1 = Less than $20,000
2 = $20,000 to $29,999
3 = $30,000 to $39,999
4 = $40,000 to $49,999
5 = $50,000 to $59,999
6 = $60,000 to $74,999
7 = $75,000 or more

17. Are you employed outside the home? *(Please circle your response.)*
1 = Yes
2 = No

18. Do you have access to the Internet either at home or at work?
(Please circle your response.)
1 = Yes
2 = No

19. Any suggestions or comments?
_____
_____
_____

Name _____
Address _____
_____

TOTAL BODY GUIDE

FROM THE EDITORS OF *PREVENTION* MAGAZINE

RODALE

TOTAL BODY GUIDE

© 2003 by Rodale Inc.
Photography credits appear on p. 184.

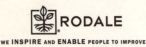

RODALE

WE INSPIRE AND ENABLE PEOPLE TO IMPROVE THEIR LIVES AND THE WORLD AROUND THEM

FOR PRODUCTS & INFORMATION
WWW.RODALESTORE.COM
WWW.PREVENTION.COM
(800) 848-4735

WOMEN'S HEALTH TOTAL BODY GUIDE STAFF

EDITOR: **Selene Yeager**

DESIGNER: **Rita Baker**

PHOTO EDITOR: **Stephanie Imhoff**

EDITORIAL RESEARCHER: **Amy Jo Van Bodegraven**

COPY EDITOR: **D. J. Caruso**

LAYOUT DESIGNER: **Jennifer H. Giandomenico**

PRODUCT SPECIALIST: **Jodi Schaffer**

RODALE WOMEN'S HEALTH GROUP

PRESIDENT, WOMEN'S PUBLISHING GROUP: **Sara Levinson**

PREVENTION EDITOR-IN-CHIEF: **Catherine Cassidy**

EDITOR-IN-CHIEF, WOMEN'S HEALTH BOOKS: **Tammerly Booth**

PREVENTION SPECIAL INTEREST PUBLICATIONS
EXECUTIVE EDITOR: **Cindi Caciolo**

DIRECT RESPONSE MARKETING

VICE PRESIDENT, PUBLISHER: **Gregg Michaelson**

DIRECTOR, PRODUCT MARKETING: **Janine Slaughter**

RODALE RETAIL SALES (800) 845-8050

RETAIL MARKETING MANAGER: **Mark Buckalew**

DIRECTOR OF DIRECT STORE DELIVERY: **Phil Trinkle**

ADVERTISING SALES

VICE PRESIDENT, PUBLISHER: **Denise Favorule**

NATIONAL ADVERTISING DIRECTOR: **Bob Ziltz**

NATIONAL ADVERTISING MANAGER: **Toni Schaller**

ADVERTISING PRODUCTION COORDINATOR: **Charlie Luecke**

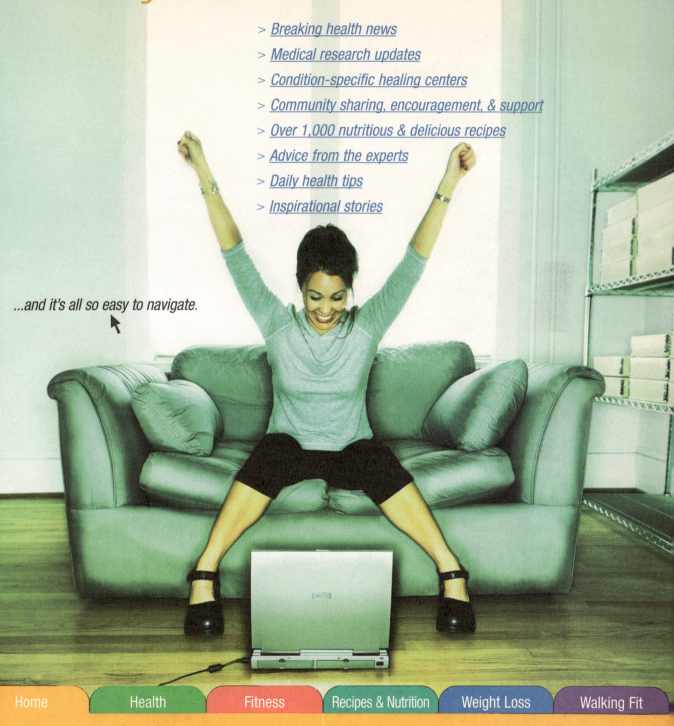

Finally!

Everything you're looking for in health is in site.

> *Breaking health news*
> *Medical research updates*
> *Condition-specific healing centers*
> *Community sharing, encouragement, & support*
> *Over 1,000 nutritious & delicious recipes*
> *Advice from the experts*
> *Daily health tips*
> *Inspirational stories*

...and it's all so easy to navigate.

| Home | Health | Fitness | Recipes & Nutrition | Weight Loss | Walking Fit |

newsite. **new**tools. all**health.** all**the time.**

PREVENTION.COM
We Help People Enjoy Healthier Lives

contents

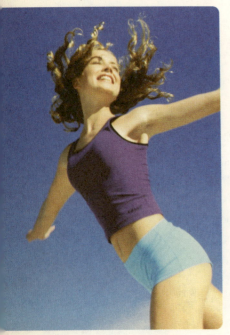

p. 26
Firmer,
smoother legs
are yours!

INTRODUCTION
1   Finally, a Get-Fit Plan You Can Really Live With!

PART **ONE**
get firm fast!

CHAPTER **1**
4   Tone It Up!
Strength training: the jumping-off point to your best body ever.

CHAPTER **2**
12   Core Moves for Fab Abs
Try these cutting-edge exercises for a tight, toned midsection.

CHAPTER **3**
20   Tone on the Go
Hit the road with this 10-minute total-body workout to stay fit anytime, anywhere!

CHAPTER **4**
26   Lower-Body Cellulite Blitz
Banish annoying lumps and bumps in just 20 minutes!

CHAPTER **5**
32   Upper-Body Beautiful
Arm yourself for sleeveless styles with these torso-toning moves.

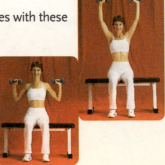

p. 36
Sexy shoulders
in one move!

SHOP *PREVENTION*

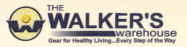

THE WALKER'S warehouse
Gear for Healthy Living...Every Step of the Way

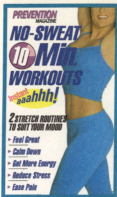

No-Sweat 10 Min. Workouts!

Two stretch routines to help you feel younger, more energized, and more flexible

ITEM	NUMBER	PRICE	QTY.	TOTAL
	RD-4015	$15.95		
Digital Step Pedometer The easiest way to walk off weight	RD-5000	~~$26.95~~ $21.95		
PREVENTION's All-Time Best Weight Loss Plan An inspiring planner, proven advice, and more than 90 delicious recipes guaranteed to slim you down! (2 books)	RD-4025	$17.95		
Outsmart Diabetes This 208-page publication will put you in charge of your diabetes instead of letting it control you!	RD-4023	$15.95		
PREVENTION's Fat to Fit Our energizing aerobic workout video for all levels	RD-4002	$15.95		
PREVENTION's Fat to Firm in 20 Minutes! A total-body, strength training workout video	RD-4001	$15.95		
Fit & Firm Pregnancy A total-body workout video for moms-to-be. Double your energy, ease back pain, and feel great!	RD-4016	$15.95		

FOR ORDERS ONLY,
CALL (800) 325-3186

Subtotal	$
S&H Charge (1st item)	$ 3.00
S&H for additional items ($1 each) _____ Items X $1.00	$
(FL residents, please include applicable sales tax)	$
TOTAL (US Dollars)	$

PAYMENT METHOD

☐ **Check or Money Order**

☐ **Visa**   ☐ **Mastercard**

☐ **Amex**   ☐ **Discover**

CREDIT CARD #

_____

EXP. DATE ___ ___ ___ ___

ORDERED BY (PLEASE PRINT)

Name _____

Address _____

City _____ **State** _____ **Zip** _____

Cardholder's Signature _____

Please make your check or money order payable to **The Walker's Warehouse.** Send this form (or a copy) and your payment to The Walker's Warehouse, Dept. 16, 304 Tequesta Dr., Tequesta, FL 33469. Allow 3 to 4 weeks for delivery. Thank you!

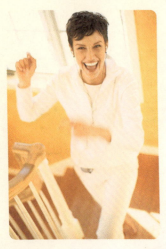

p. 42
Take the "work"
out of workout.

PART **TWO**
cardio blast!

CHAPTER **6**
40 5 Steps to Cardio Success
Turn on your fat burners with these workout tips.

CHAPTER **7**
47 Personalize Your Cardio Plan
Discover the workouts that are perfect for your personality
and lifestyle.

CHAPTER **8**
51 Blast Fat to the Max!
Kick your body-toning plan into high gear with these
fat-burning exercises.

PART **THREE**
stretch it out!

CHAPTER **9**
66 Tone Up and Get Flexible Fast
Stretch out your fitness benefits with this daily routine.

CHAPTER **10**
74 Essential Stretches for Stress Relief
These fluid moves will help you stand up straight with
a smile.

CHAPTER **11**
78 7 Moves to a More Balanced You
Ease achy muscles and an anxious mind with this
ancient discipline.

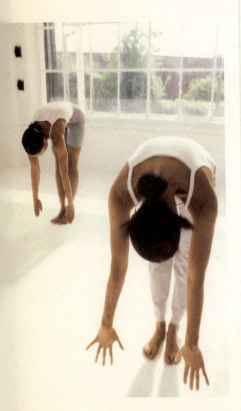

p. 66
Feel-good moves
for a great-
looking body.

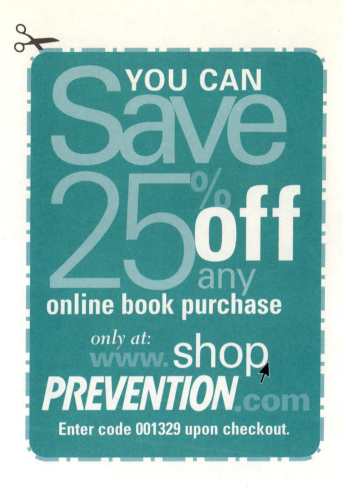

YOU CAN
Save
25%off
any
online book purchase

only at:
www.shop
PREVENTION.com

Enter code 001329 upon checkout.

Valid on ShopPrevention.com online orders only.
Coupon may not be combined with other discount offers or used more than once.
Cannot be applied to existing orders.
Offer expires February 28, 2004.

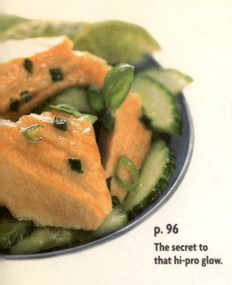

p. 96
The secret to
that hi-pro glow.

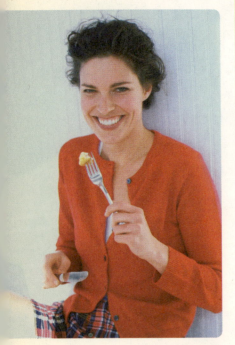

p. 100
Losing weight doesn't mean
depriving yourself.

PART **FOUR**
eat to lose!

CHAPTER **12**
86 Sorting Out the Carb Confusion
Low-carbohydrate eating made safe, fast, and easy!

CHAPTER **13**
96 Pick Your Protein Wisely
Smart cuts can make meat a healthy and tasty part of
your weight loss plan.

CHAPTER **14**
100 Welcome Back Fat!
The savory flavors you love can *finally* be part of a
healthy weight loss diet!

CHAPTER **15**
104 Customize Your Weight Loss Plan
Get the body you've always wanted eating foods you love.

PART **FIVE**
real meals you'll love

CHAPTER **16**
110 7 Days to a Slimmer You
An easy-to-follow meal plan to start you on the road
to low-carb success.

CHAPTER **17**
122 Start the Day the Smart Low-Carb Way
These quick and yummy morning meals will get your
day—and diet—started off in the right direction.

CHAPTER **18**
128 Real Power Lunches
Try these easy-to-make, high-protein dishes for fast and
slimming midday meals.

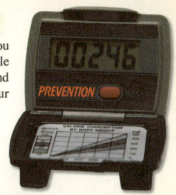
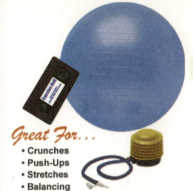 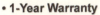
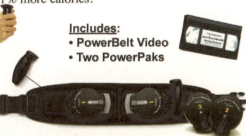
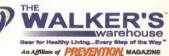

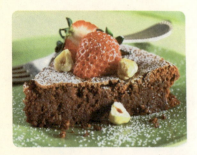

p. 152
Chocolate Hazelnut Flourless Cake.

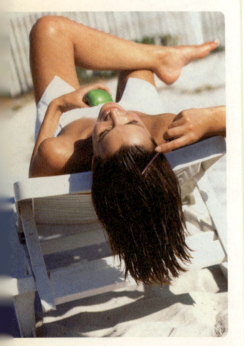

p. 176
Be the mane event with a new style.

CHAPTER **19**

134 Savory Dinners

One bite of these filling, flavorful dishes, and you'll never look at low-carb the same way again.

CHAPTER **20**

145 Just Desserts

These yummy treats prove that low-carb dieters can have their cake (and pudding and cookies) and their waistline too.

PART **SIX**

keep the drive alive!

CHAPTER **21**

156 17 Tips for Putting You First

Here's how to work out without stressing yourself (and your family and your boss) out.

CHAPTER **22**

162 10 Gotta-Have Workout Toys

New exercise gadgets can be fun, motivational, and may even help keep you safe.

CHAPTER **23**

165 Workouts to Match Your Mood

Don't let your emotional ups and downs sabotage your fitness.

PART **SEVEN**

bonus beauty section!

CHAPTER **24**

170 Get Glowing from Head to Toe

A no-fail regimen for rejuvenating your on-the-go skin.

CHAPTER **25**

176 Crowning Glory: Here's to Hair!

The right cut, color, and style can carry you from flabby to fabulous.

CHAPTER **26**

180 Dress for Exercise Success

This activewear will keep you going and going and going!

Finally, a Get-Fit Plan You Can Really Live With!

I'm here to give you some good news. Some really good news. The face of fitness has changed. And it's a whole lot brighter and prettier than it used to be. Remember those piles of pasta we used to call "diet food"? Gone. Those manic, high-impact, "feel the burn" aerobics classes we swore by? Gone too. In their place, we have a smart, low-carb diet bursting with veggies, fruits, whole grains, healthy fats, and protein, and a fitness regimen that rolls fat-blasting cardio, muscle-toning strength training, and mind/body exercise into one balanced plan. It's sensible. It's doable. Most importantly, it works.

Now, here's some even better news. We at *Prevention* have put all of this cutting-edge diet and exercise advice together in the *Total Body Guide* you're holding in your hands. In it, we bring you exercises that really flatten your abs fast without a single crunch. We tell you which cardio melts fat fastest. We sort out the maddening carbohydrate confusion. We even give you real-life tips for starting—and sticking with—a diet and exercise program in the midst of your already hectic life.

You'll also find an entire section filled with great-tasting, easy-to-make recipes for breakfast through dinner, plus dessert (yes, including chocolate!). Just one bite, and you'll quickly see that low-carb doesn't have to mean low satisfaction! Because we know that every woman wants to look great as well as feel great, we've also added a bonus beauty section, complete with advice from the top US skin, hair, and image pros that will have you looking fashion forward without breaking your budget.

At *Prevention*, we realize that there are a gazillion books, magazines, and Internet sites doling out conflicting, sometimes confusing, health and fitness information. That's why we handpicked all the real advice you need to finally get the body you want in the time you have. Opening this book is the first step to getting in the best shape of your life. I, for one, plan to get cracking right away!

Catherine Cassidy
Editor-in-Chief
Prevention Magazine

part 1

get firm fast!

4 **Tone It Up!**
Strength training: the jumping-off point
to your best body ever

12 **Core Moves for Fab Abs**
Try these cutting-edge exercises for a tight,
toned midsection

20 **Tone on the Go**
Hit the road with this 10-minute total-body workout
to stay fit anytime, anywhere!

26 **Lower-Body Cellulite Blitz**
Banish annoying lumps and bumps in just 20 minutes!

32 **Upper-Body Beautiful**
Arm yourself for sleeveless styles with these
torso-toning moves

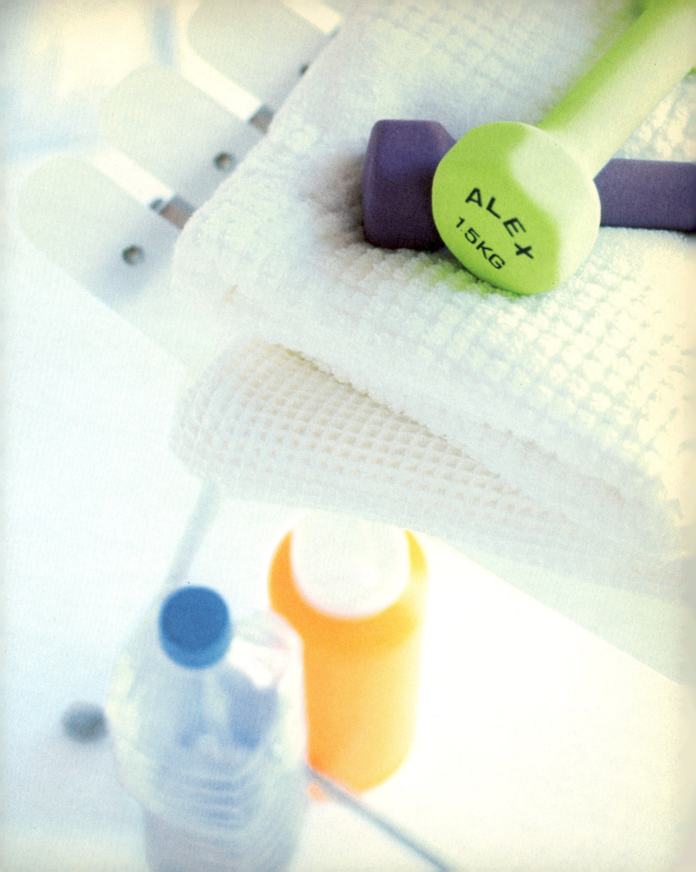

CHAPTER 1

Tone It Up!

Strength training: the jumping-off point to your best body ever

It happens to the best of us. One day we wake up and, suddenly, giving up chocolate for a few days or adding an extra aerobics class or two during the week just won't get rid of those stubborn pounds. It's not your imagination. Losing weight gets a little harder each year. But it's not impossible! With the right kind of workout—and we'll give you a hint, it's *not* cardio—you can burn up to 200 extra calories a day, many of them while doing nothing more challenging than watching your favorite movie or eating dinner. The result: You could lose up to 20 lb in a year—without eating less.

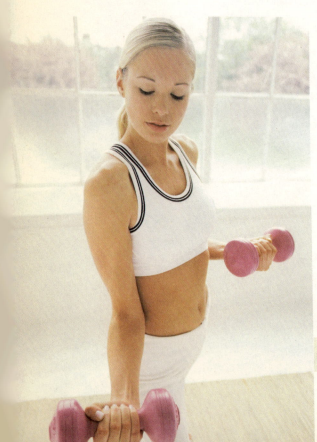

Work your arms to trim your waist.

Master Your Metabolism

Metabolism is all the work your body does that requires calories (energy): staying alive, thinking, breathing, and moving your muscles. Obviously, it plays a major role in how much you weigh, especially with each passing birthday.

Sometime in your 30s, your metabolism starts slowing down by about 5% every decade. That means if you eat about 1,800 calories a day and fit into size 10s when you're 35, you'll be shopping for 12s when you're 45, even if you're eating the same number of calories. By the time you're 55, well, you get the idea.

The culprit behind this decline in calorie-burn is muscle loss, says Steve Farrell, PhD, associate director of The Cooper Institute in Dallas. Every pound of muscle you lose can decrease the number of calories you burn by as many as 30 a day. In the years before menopause, you start losing about 1/2 lb of muscle a year, a loss that can double once you hit menopause (blame it on lack of activity and just plain aging). If you're not careful, by the time you're 65, it's possible to have lost half of your muscle mass and see your metabolism slowed by 200 to 300 calories.

Firm and Burn!

To keep your metabolism chugging in high gear, you need strength training. If you work your major muscle groups twice a week, you can expect to replace 5 to 10 years' worth of muscle loss in just a few months. Lifting weights can literally reverse the aging process, so you look and feel years, maybe even decades, younger.

Lifting weights increases your calorie-burn in other ways too. In one study, 15 sedentary people in their 60s and 70s who strength trained 3 days a

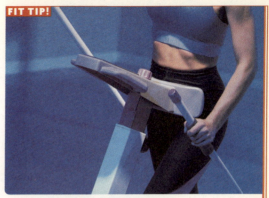

FIT TIP!

Master the machines
If balance or coordination is a problem during strength training, try working out on resistance machines (such as Nautilus) at your gym. They restrict your range of motion, so it's easier to perform moves correctly.

week for 6 months increased their daily calorie-burn by more than 230 calories. Almost one-third of the increase was from a boost in their metabolism due to the muscle they gained. The remaining calories were burned as a result of their workouts, their increased daily activity, and something called "afterburn," which is an added attraction of strength training exercise. Depending on how hard you work out, explains study author Gary R. Hunter, PhD, of the University of Alabama at Birmingham, your metabolism can stay elevated for up to 48 hours after you've finished lifting.

"As a bonus, strength training builds bone," says Dr. Farrell. That's important because after menopause, women can lose up to 20% of their bone strength. "Though we tend to think of bones as 'dead,' they are very alive and highly active. Strong bones use more nutrients, and ultimately they burn more calories than do weak bones," he explains.

The Rev-It-Up Routine

To make things easy, we've created a customized strength training plan for women. Do 10 to 12 repetitions of each exercise. Rest for 30 to 60 seconds between exercises. Do this workout three times a week, allowing a day of rest in between. For best results, use an amount of weight that will be difficult to lift during your last few reps.

PLIÉ

Stand with your feet about 2 feet apart; your legs should be turned out. With your back straight, lower your body. Then, as you straighten your legs, squeeze your inner thighs. Your knees should be in line with your ankles. Return to the starting position. Hold dumbbells to make the move more challenging.

[1]

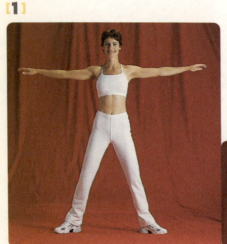

[2]

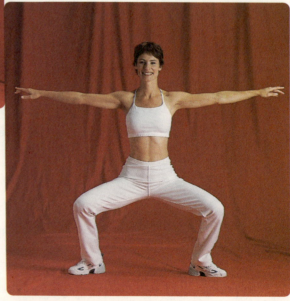

LUNGE

Lightly place your left hand on the back of a chair for balance. Step forward with your left foot. Your knee should be above your left foot, not sticking out past your toes. Lower your body by bending your knees and dropping your hips straight toward the floor. Return to the starting position, then repeat with the other leg. To make it more challenging, do the move without the chair, and hold dumbbells down at your sides.

[1]

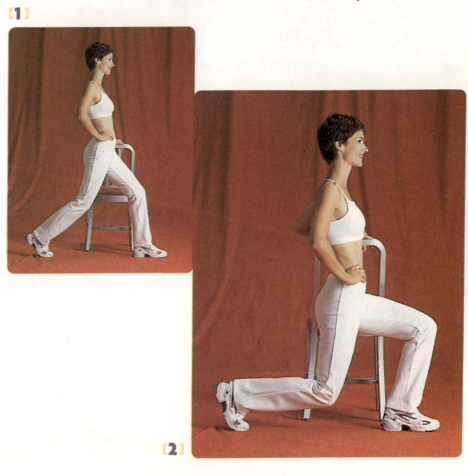

[2]

SEATED LEG LIFT

Place ankle weights around each ankle. Sit in a chair with your knees bent 90 degrees and your feet flat on the floor. Slowly lift your lower left leg until it is in line with your thigh. Slowly lower. Repeat with your right leg.

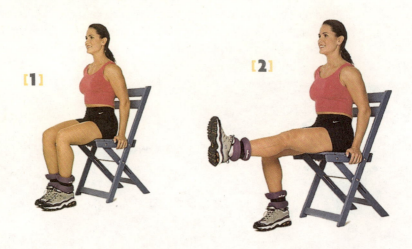

HAMSTRING CURL

Place ankle weights around each ankle. Lie facedown on the floor (you can place a pillow under your hips for comfort). Place your arms under your head, and rest your head on your forearms. Bending your left knee, bring your foot toward your butt until your leg is bent at a 90-degree angle. Keep your hips on the floor and your foot flexed. Slowly lower. Repeat with your right leg.

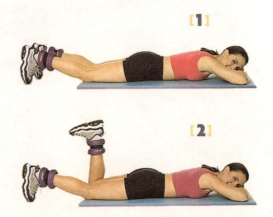

PULLOVER

Lie on a mat or a weight bench. Grasp a dumbbell with both hands, and hold it above your chest. Without bending your elbows, lower it backward over your head as far as comfortably possible. Don't arch your back. Slowly return to the starting position.

[1]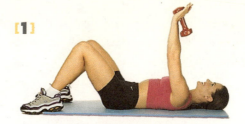

[2]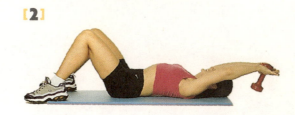

DO JUST ONE THING!

Knock out joint pain

Lifting weights shouldn't hurt. If it does, you may just need to adjust your form, says Reebok trainer Joy Prouty of Palm Beach, FL. Here's what she recommends for common exercise "ouches."

EXERCISE	COMPLAINT	THE FIX
Chest press	Shoulder pain	Do the exercise on the floor, so your elbows cannot dip lower than your shoulders. Or try kneeling push-ups, without touching your chest to the floor.
Lunge	Knee pain	Step back into lunges, instead of forward. You're less likely to pitch your weight too far over your knee.
Lateral raise	Shoulder pain	Raise your arms slightly in front of you to form a big V, instead of lifting straight out to the side. Don't lift higher than your shoulders.
Overhead press	Shoulder pain	Start with your palms facing your ears (instead of forward), and point your elbows slightly forward.

The Rev-It-Up Routine

CHEST FLY

Lie on a mat or a weight bench. Hold dumbbells above your chest with your palms facing each other and your elbows slightly bent. Slowly lower your arms out to the sides, then raise them.

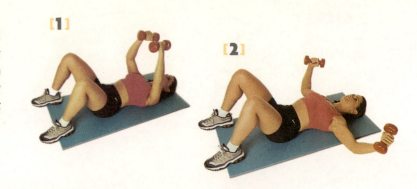

TRICEPS KICKBACK

Put your right hand on a bench or chair, keeping your back flat. Hold a dumbbell with your left arm bent at a 90-degree angle and your elbow at your side. Lifting the dumbbell backward, extend your arm until it is straight. Don't move your upper arm or shoulder. Slowly lower. Repeat with your right arm.

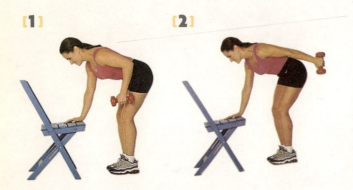

REVERSE CURL

Lie on your back on a mat, arms down at your sides. Bend your hips and knees so that your legs are over your midsection and relaxed. Slowly contract your abdominal muscles, lifting your hips about 2 to 4 inches off the floor. Slowly lower.

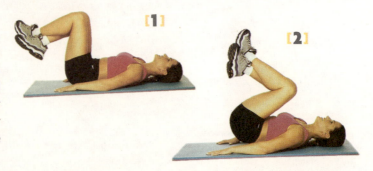

DIAGONAL CURL-UP

Lie on your back on a mat. Clasp your hands lightly behind your head. Slowly lift your head and shoulders off the floor, twist to the left, and bring your right shoulder toward your left knee. Slowly lower. Repeat, alternating sides.

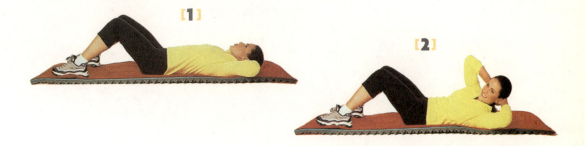

If you work your major muscle groups twice a week, you can expect to replace 5 to 10 years' worth of muscle loss in just a few months.

CALF RAISE

Stand with your feet about hip-width apart, holding dumbbells at your sides. Slowly rise up onto your toes while keeping your torso and legs straight. Hold, then lower.

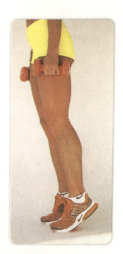

CHAPTER 2

Core Moves for Fab Abs

Try these cutting-edge exercises for a tight, toned midsection

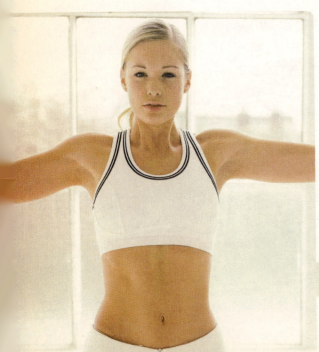

Even more than toned hips and thighs, women want firm, flat abs to show off in today's body-hugging styles. And they think the road to an iron middle is paved with hundreds and hundreds of crunches. Well, crunch time is over! The new breed of belly toners challenges your abdominal muscles while working your entire torso and "core" (back, abs, hips, and pelvis), giving you fast, visible results, as well as greater strength and stability to do all the sports and activities you love.

The new ab exercises make your abs work to stabilize your body. This recruits and tones more deep abdominal muscle fibers

Strengthen your foundation to get flat and firm.

than ordinary crunches, says New York City–based trainer Liz Neporent, who teaches Quick Fix Ab Training, a 15-minute "crunchless" class. "Crunches can be effective, but they're not the only way to work your abs," says Neporent. "There are too many ways to cheat on crunches without even knowing it, such as by pulling on your head or using your hip flexors instead of your abs. These new moves are not only effective for your abs, but they also strengthen your back, butt, and arms."

Catherine Samuels, 38-year-old mother of three, couldn't agree more. "Now, my whole core is tighter and stronger," says Samuels, who never worked her abs before because she thought crunches were useless. "These moves work so well that 2 weeks after my youngest son was born, my belly was flat, and I was wearing a belt!"

The Crunchless Fab-Ab Plan

Do one to three sets of 8 to 15 repetitions of each exercise (unless otherwise specified) 2 or 3 days a week, avoiding back-to-back days. The entire workout will take less than 15 minutes. You'll feel straighter and stronger in as little as a week. You'll see definite results in 4 to 6 weeks.

HOVER

Lie facedown on the floor with your upper body propped on your forearms and your elbows directly beneath your shoulders. Your torso should be off the floor so your body is in a straight line. Don't let your belly droop. Hold for 10 to 20 seconds. One rep is enough. If you have back problems, skip this move.

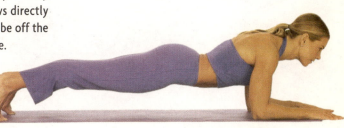

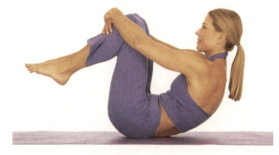

ROLL-LIKE-A-BALL

Sit on the floor, and hug your knees to your chest. Balance on your tailbone, and lift your feet, pointing your toes toward the floor. Pull your ab muscles in, and roll back onto your lower back. Contract your abs, and pull yourself back to the starting position. If the move is too difficult, loosen your arms, so your knees are pulled less tightly to your body.

BICYCLE

Lie faceup on the floor, with your legs extended and your hands loosely behind your head. Slowly bring your right elbow across your body while bending your left knee and lifting your leg toward your chest as far as comfortably possible. Hold, then lower. Repeat, alternating sides. You should be twisting your torso, not your neck.

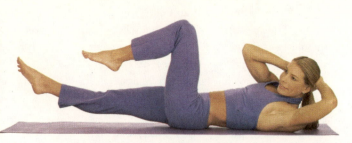

BALL PUSH-UP

Lie facedown on an exercise ball with your hands on the floor. Walk your hands out until the ball is under your shins (or under your thighs to make it easier). Your hands should be directly beneath your shoulders. Keeping your torso straight and your abs contracted, bend your elbows, lowering your chest toward the floor until your upper arms are parallel to the floor. Pause, then push back up.

DO JUST ONE THING!

Abs first!

Short on exercise time? Work your abs! In a 13-year study of more than 8,100 people, Canadian researchers found that those with the strongest abs (measured by how many sit-ups they could perform) were significantly less likely to die during the study period than those who had the weakest abs. Why? Scientists believe strong abs mean more calorie-burning muscle tissue and less belly fat, which in turn can lower your risk of diabetes and heart disease. A flat, strong tummy can also make performing everyday tasks easier, so you stay mobile and independent longer.

FIT TIP!   Straighten up

All the ab exercises in the world are worthless if you have droopy posture. To stand and sit straighter, tighten your abs just enough that your hips are straight under your body and your shoulders are slightly back and in line. That's how your abs should always feel.

SIDE PLANK

Lie on your side with your upper body propped on your left elbow and forearm. Put your right hand on your hip. Pressing into your left forearm, raise your hips and thighs off the floor so your body forms a straight line. Hold for 5 seconds, then switch sides.

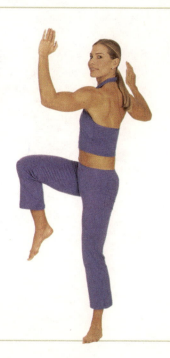

STANDING CROSSOVER

Stand with your feet a few inches apart. Bend your arms, and hold them out to your sides so they form right angles with your fingertips, palms facing forward. Contract your abs, and pull your right knee and left elbow toward one another. Pause, then return to the starting position. Complete a set, then switch sides.

Shoot for Six

These moves will rock your rectus abdominis for a sculpted, showoff-able 6-pack

That rippled midsection muscle you see peeking out from billboards and fitness mags is the rectus abdominis, the longest and most prominent of the abdominal muscle family. It's the one to target when you want sharp, sexy definition. Here are four moves that can get the job done. For the best benefits, do 2 or 3 sets of 12 reps. (Note: If you experience back pain while doing any of these exercises, stop, and check with your doctor before continuing.)

LEG RAISE

Lie on the floor, and raise your legs straight up. Place an exercise ball between your knees, then do a slight pelvic tilt from the hips. Squeeze the exercise ball for 1 second, then relax.

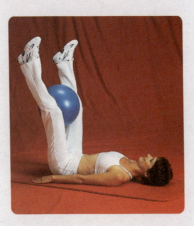

PELVIC TILT

Lie on the floor with your arms at your sides, knees bent, and feet flat on the floor. Press your lower back to the floor so that your pelvis tilts upward. Straighten your legs by slowly sliding your heels along the floor, and stop when you can no longer hold a full tilt position; hold for a count of six. Next, move one leg at a time back to the starting position, maintaining the pelvic tilt throughout. Hold the starting position for six counts, then relax.

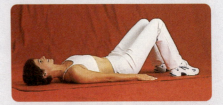

SEATED BODY LIFT

Sit erect in a firm, armless chair, and place your hands on the sides of the chair in front of your hips. Tighten your abs, and support yourself with your hands as you slowly pull your knees up toward your chest. Keep your lower back against the chair back. Hold, then slowly lower. (This move is more easily performed without shoes.)

HIP RAISE

Lie on the floor, and place an exercise ball between your bent knees. Lift your hips off the floor, and bring your knees toward your chest. Squeeze the ball for 1 second, then relax.

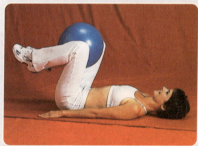

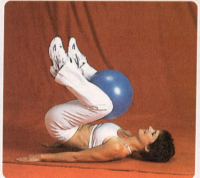

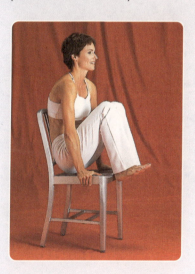

FIT TIP! Try an instant belly toner

Do this core move anywhere: Sit with your hand on your stomach. Inhale through your nose for 4 seconds. Hold for 7 seconds, then exhale for 8 seconds. Feel your hand rise and fall. Repeat.

Get Ballerina Beautiful

Try these classic dancer moves for a stronger, leaner core

Dancers know that the secret to a lean, beautiful body is a well-toned "core" (back, abdomen, hips, and pelvis). So they developed their own special exercises to keep theirs firm and fat-free. Try these moves to improve your posture and erase that stubborn lower-belly pouch. These exercises will also protect your back from pain and injury, says Peggy W. Brill, a physical therapist and author of *The Core Program* (BantamDoubleday, 2003).

Do these sample exercises 5 days a week. Stretch afterward.

BUTTERFLY & HEEL BEAT

Lie facedown, arms at your sides, palms up. Tighten your abs by pushing your pubic bone to the floor, and squeeze your shoulder blades together, lifting your chest as high as possible and raising your arms up to your buttocks. Hold for 6 seconds, then lower. Immediately fold your arms beneath your head, lift your legs up to buttock level, and open your feet wider than shoulder-width, toes out. Click your heels together repeatedly for a count of 20. Return to the starting position. Repeat for three sets of butterflies and two sets of heel beats.

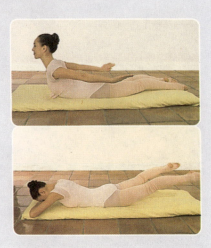

TURN UP THE BURN!

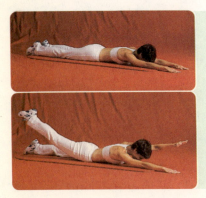

Support your spine

A strong back is the perfect posture-improving complement to toned abs. This easy back-strengthener can help.

Lie facedown with your legs extended straight behind you, toes pointed, and arms extended straight in front of you. Keep your chin up off the floor at a comfortable level. Slowly raise your left arm and your right leg at the same time until they are both a few inches off the floor. Hold, then slowly lower them back to the starting position. Repeat with the opposite arm and leg.

DEAD BUG

Lie on your back, knees bent. Press the small of your back to the floor, tighten your abs, and straighten your arms toward the ceiling, with your hands making fists and your thumbs pointing overhead. Holding your abs tight, alternate dropping one arm overhead toward the floor and the other toward your knees as many times as possible to a count of 30. Return to the starting posi-

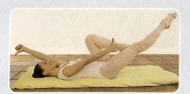

tion, and bring your knees toward your chest. Straighten your right leg to 45 degrees from the floor, pull it back in, then repeat with the left. Alternate for a count of 30. Now combine both motions, so that when one leg moves toward your chest, the arm on the same side is reaching overhead. Alternate to a count of 60.

PELVIC STABILIZER

Lie on your right side, propped on your right forearm with your abs tight. Stack your legs, and place them straight out at a 45-degree angle. Keeping your feet flexed, lift your top leg 3 inches, and kick it forward as far as possible. Repeat six times, then kick backward six times without arching your back. Finally, rotate the top leg so your toes point to the ceiling, and circle it clockwise. Then circle it counter-clockwise six times. Repeat with the other leg.

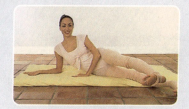

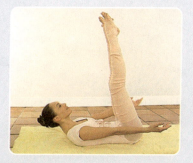

MERMAID

Lie on your back with your legs straight up at a 90-degree angle, toes pointing slightly out. Place your arms at your sides, palms up. Press your back to the floor, and lift your head and upper back as high as possible, raising your arms to hip level. Pulse your arms up and down to a count of six, breathing in, then turn your palms down, and pulse again to a six count, breathing out. Repeat six times.

CHAPTER 3

Tone on the Go

Hit the road with this 10-minute total-body workout to stay fit anytime, anywhere!

Just because your busy life has you in a constant state of "on the go" doesn't mean you have to put your fitness goals in a permanent holding pattern. With just 10 minutes and an exercise band, you can squeeze in a total-body toning workout no matter where your hectic life takes you. This very simple routine firms and sculpts almost all your major muscles. It's such a breeze that you'll never miss a workout again!

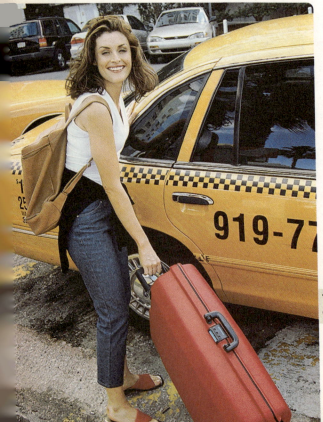

Take your workout on the road.

The Workout

For all exercises, allow about 9 seconds for each repetition (4 seconds to lift or contract, hold for 1 second, then 4 seconds to lower or extend). Do 10 repetitions of each exercise. If you have extra time, go for a second set for even better results.

ONE-LEG LUNGE

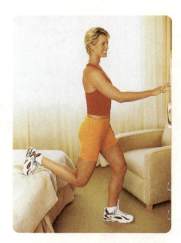

Stand with your back to a bed or chair, and place your right foot on it. Hold on to something sturdy for support. Slowly lower yourself by bending your left knee. Make sure you can always see the toes on your left foot. If you can't, move forward so that your knee stays behind your toes when you bend. Hold, then slowly come back up. Repeat with your right leg.

With just 10 minutes and an exercise band, you can squeeze in a total-body toning workout no matter where your hectic life takes you.

PUSH-UP

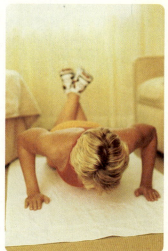

Lie on your stomach on top of a towel or blanket with your knees bent, ankles crossed, and hands by your shoulders. As you press into the floor and straighten your arms, slowly lift your chest, hips, and thighs. Hold, then slowly lower. Before you touch the floor, push up again. To make the move tougher, keep your legs straight.

BACK EXTENSION

Lying on your stomach, place your hands under your chin. Keeping your feet on the floor, slowly lift your head and chest about 3 to 5 inches. Hold, then slowly lower.

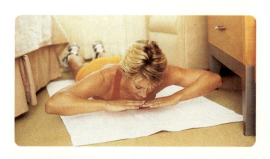

CRUNCH

Lie on your back with your knees bent, feet flat on the floor, and hands behind your head. Pressing your lower back to the floor, slowly lift your head, shoulders, and upper back. Hold, then slowly lower.

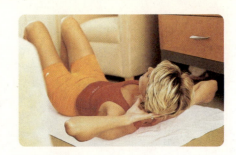

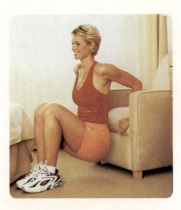

CHAIR DIP

Sitting on the edge of a chair, place your hands on the edge by your butt. (Make sure the chair is stable and won't slide out from under you.) Move your feet a few steps forward so your butt is off the chair and your knees are bent at 90-degree angles. Bending your elbows so they point behind you, lower yourself as far as comfortable. Hold, then slowly press back up.

For the following exercises, use an exercise band.

TRICEPS EXTENSION

With a towel around your neck, drape the band over the back of your neck, and bend your arms to hold the band near your chest. Keeping your elbows at your sides, straighten your arms. Hold, then slowly release.

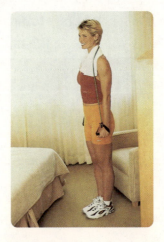

LATERAL RAISE

Sitting on a chair, place the end of the band under or around your right foot, and hold the other end in your right hand with your arm down at your side. Keeping a slight bend in your elbow, slowly lift your right arm out to the side until it's about shoulder height. Hold, then slowly lower. Repeat with your left arm.

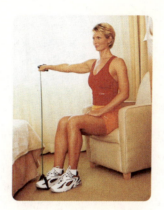

FIT TIP! **Forget sitting "like a lady"**

Take a lot of long trips? Avoid crossing your legs in your seat. It shortens the leg muscles, reduces circulation, and creates an uneven weight on the hips and pelvis, which can cause workout-stopping lower-back pain.

BICEPS CURL

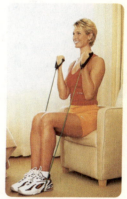

Sit on a chair with the band under both feet. With your elbows at your sides, bring your hands toward your shoulders. Hold, then slowly lower.

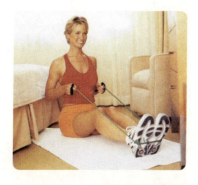

SEATED ROW

Sit on the floor with your back straight and legs out in front, knees slightly bent. Loop the band over your feet at the arches. Squeezing your shoulder blades, pull your arms back toward your chest so that your elbows are pointing behind you. Hold, then slowly release.

Twice the Toning in Half the Time!

Rev up your results with these super combo moves

Have wall-to-wall obligations left you with just 15 minutes of gym time? No sweat. Take along these superquick two-step exercises. Each move tones multiple muscles, giving you great results fast!

For best results, do 8 to 12 repetitions (per side when alternating legs), and 2 or 3 sets of each move, resting for 30 to 60 seconds between sets. Allow at least 1 day of rest between workouts.

SQUAT AND SIDE LIFT

MAJOR MUSCLES WORKED: **glutes, quads, hamstrings, outer thighs**

Wearing ankle weights, stand with your feet shoulder-width apart and your toes pointed out slightly. Keep your eyes facing forward. Bending slowly at the knees and hips, squat back as though

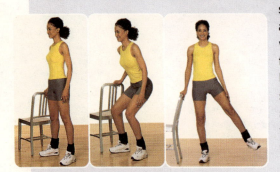

sitting in a chair. Keep your back flat, and don't allow your knees to jut over your toes. Stop when your thighs are just about parallel to the floor but not any lower. Straighten your legs, lifting your left leg off the floor and out to the side as you stand. Pause, then return to the starting position. Repeat, lifting your right leg to the side this time. Alternate legs throughout the exercise, completing a full set with each leg.

AB CURL AND CHEST PRESS

MAJOR MUSCLES WORKED: **abs, chest, triceps, shoulders**

Lie on your back with your knees bent and your feet flat on the floor. Hold a medicine ball with both hands, letting the weight rest lightly on your chest. Keep your elbows out to the sides. Tilt your pelvis slightly to keep your back flat against the floor.

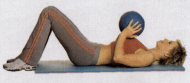

All in one move, contract your chest muscles, and straighten your arms, pushing the ball up above your chest. At the same time, contract your abdominal muscles, lifting your head and shoulders off the floor about 30 degrees. Hold, then lower the ball back down to your body, and at the same time lower your head and shoulders to the floor. Don't have a medicine ball? You can use a dumbbell instead. Just hold it by the ends.

CURL AND PRESS

MAJOR MUSCLES WORKED: **shoulders, biceps, upper back, triceps**

Sit on a sturdy chair with your feet flat on the floor. Hold a dumbbell in each hand with your arms extended down at your sides and your palms facing forward. Your back should be straight and your eyes facing forward.

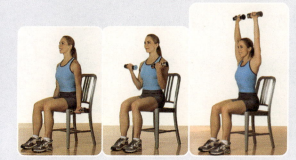

Keeping your upper body stable, bend your elbows, and curl the weights up toward your shoulders. Without hesitating, rotate your wrists so your palms are facing out in front of you. Press the weights over your head. Maintain the same distance between the dumbbells as you lift. Stop just before your arms are completely straight. The weights should be overhead and slightly in front of your body. Pause, slowly reverse the movement, and lower the weights.

STEP AND SQUEEZE

MAJOR MUSCLES WORKED: **glutes, lower back, hamstrings, inner thighs, quads, calves**

Stand about a foot away from a step with your feet about hip-width apart. Place your hands on your hips. (You can hold light dumbbells at your hips once you get comfortable with the move.) While this exercise is demonstrated here on an aerobic step, you can use a step in your home.

Keeping your upper body straight, step forward with your left foot, placing it on the center of the step. All in one move, straighten your left leg, lift your right foot off the floor, squeeze your buttocks, and extend your right leg behind you with your toes pointed toward the floor. Pause, then raise your body up on the ball of your left foot. Hold, then slowly reverse the motion, lowering yourself onto your left foot, bringing your right leg down, and stepping back to the floor. Repeat with the opposite leg. Alternate legs until you complete a full set with each.

CHAPTER 4

Lower-Body Cellulite Blitz

Banish annoying lumps and bumps in just 20 minutes!

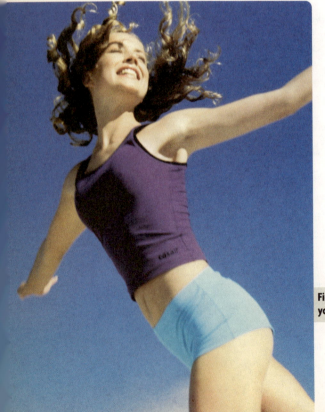

Finally, a rear view you'll love.

Finally, here's a proven answer for firmer, smoother legs. After years of dieting, slathering on globs of product, shelling out for pricey seaweed wraps and special massages, and hiding your lower half in cover-ups of all kinds, we *finally* have a plan that will help you shed cellulite once and for all. The best part: It takes only 20 minutes, 3 days a week.

With this exercise plan, you can reduce cellulite and make your lower body look smoother and firmer, says *Prevention* advisor Wayne L. Westcott, PhD, who developed our Cellulite Blitz Exercises. "When we put 16 women ages 26 to 66 on our program for 8 weeks, all of them reported less cellulite in their lower body. And 70% of them reported a lot less," he says.

It wasn't just wishful thinking. On average, the women lost just over 3 lb of fat, added 2^1/$_2$ lb of muscle, and shed almost 1^1/$_2$ inches from their hips. What's more, ultrasound tests confirmed it. Overall, the women shrank the lumpy fat layer on their thighs by 1.3 millimeters (mm) and increased smooth muscle tissue in the same area by 1.8 mm. It doesn't sound like much, but it definitely made their legs look smoother and firmer.

The Real Deal on Cellulite

The best part of this program is that it puts to rest the mistaken notion that cellulite is some mysterious female "condition." Despite what you've heard about trapped toxins or poor circulation being to blame, cellulite is one thing: fat. It just looks different because of how it's arranged.

Everyone has strands of connective tissue that separate fat cells into compartments and connect fat tissue to skin. In women, these fibers form a honeycomb-like pattern, so any increase of fat in a given area tends to bulge. You don't see cellulite in men because their fibers run in a horizontal, crisscross pattern that prevents bulging or dimpling.

So why does cellulite seem to appear out of nowhere and get worse as we get older? Two reasons. First, it's because tissue changes. Those strands of connective tissue thicken with age, and

FIT TIP! **Lose weight sensibly**
Avoid crash dieting; it can make cellulite worse. When you lose weight quickly, you lose muscle tissue—the stuff that makes your legs and butt look toned and smooth.

our skin gets thinner, says Katie Rodan, MD, clinical assistant professor of dermatology at Stanford University. "The combined effect is more pronounced cellulite," she explains.

Second, and more important, too many of us let our body composition go soft—literally—as we get older. The average woman loses 5 lb of muscle and replaces it with about 15 lb of fat every decade of her adult life, says Dr. Westcott. "Because fat is exceptionally soft, it doesn't keep our skin taut like muscle does. It also takes up more space, so it bulges out."

To get rid of cellulite, you have to reduce the underlying fat stores and replace lost muscle tissue. "You won't find a cellulite cure in cosmetic products or procedures," says Jeffrey Sklar, MD, assistant clinical professor of dermatology at Columbia University in New York City. "But the more muscle tone you have, the less of a problem it will be."

The Cellulite Blitz Program

Follow this three-step, 20-minute program 3 days a week to dump those unwanted dimples.

1. **Cardio**—Warm up with 2 minutes of moderate walking, cycling, or stairclimbing (you can use indoor stationary machines). Increase intensity for 8 minutes. Work vigorously enough to be breathing hard but still able to talk in short sentences. Lower the intensity, and cool down for 2 minutes.

2. Strength—Do one set of 10 to 15 repetitions of each of the exercises, using a weight that's heavy enough to fatigue your muscles. (This is essential for optimum muscle building in these areas.) Your muscles are fatigued when you feel as though you can't do even one more repetition. When you can easily complete 15 reps, increase the weight slightly. Work slowly, counting 2 seconds to lift and 4 seconds to lower.

3. Flexibility—After each strength training exercise, you need to stretch the muscle you just worked. Do each stretch once, holding for 20 seconds. Dr. Westcott has found that adopting this stretching strategy can boost strength training results by 20%.

The Cellulite Blitz Exercises

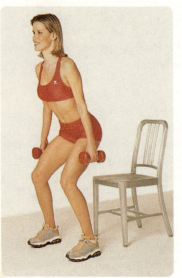

DUMBBELL SQUAT ➤

Stand with your back to a chair and your feet about shoulder-width apart. Hold dumbbells down by your sides, palms facing in. Keeping your back straight, bend from the knees and hips as though you are sitting down. Don't let your knees move forward over your toes. Stop just shy of touching the chair, then stand back up.

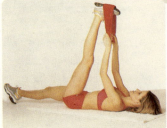

◄ **Follow with a Lying Hamstring Stretch**
Lying faceup with legs extended, use a towel or rope to pull each leg in toward your chest. Don't lock your knee.

The Cellulite Blitz Exercises

LUNGE ➤

Standing with your feet together, hold dumbbells down at your sides with palms facing in. Take one big step forward with your right leg. Plant your right foot, then slowly lower your left knee toward the floor. Your right knee should be bent at a 90-degree angle and your back straight. Press into your right foot, and push yourself back to the starting position. Repeat with your left leg.

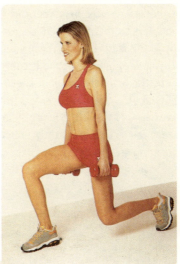

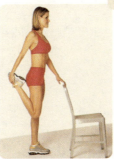

◄ **Follow with a Standing Quadriceps Stretch**
Standing straight, gently pull your right foot toward your butt. Repeat with your left leg.

The average woman loses 5 lb of muscle and replaces it with about 15 lb of fat every decade of her adult life.

The Cellulite Blitz Exercises

INNER THIGH PRESS ▶

Lie faceup with your arms at your sides. Bend your knees slightly, and raise your legs so they form a 90-degree angle with your body. (If this is too difficult, bend your knees more, and lift your legs only as high as is comfortable.) Place an exercise ball between your knees; your feet should be flexed. Slowly squeeze your legs together against the resistance of the ball as hard as you can, making sure to keep your knees bent slightly. When the resistance becomes too great to press any farther, hold for 3 seconds. Then slowly open back to the starting position.

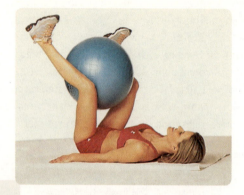

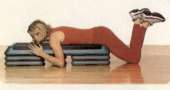

◀ **Follow with a Butterfly Stretch**
Sitting with the soles of your feet together, place your hands on the top of your inner thighs, knees out to the sides, and lean forward from the hips.

TURN UP THE BURN!

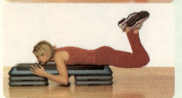

Build a killer booty

For most women, their butt is their cellulite sore spot. This Glute Buster is a killer move for building those butt muscles and tightening up a lumpy rear view. Bonus: This move also strengthens your back. Do one to three sets of 8 to 12 reps the same day you do the Cellulite Blitz Program.

Lie facedown on an aerobic step or bench with your legs hanging down off the end and your hips bent at a 45- to 90-degree angle. Bend your knees, and cross your ankles. Hold on to the edges of the step for support. Keep your head down.

Tighten your abs to help support your lower back. Keeping your knees bent, slowly lift your legs until your thighs are in line with your body and are parallel to the floor, but not higher. Pause, then slowly lower back to the starting position.

SCISSORS PRESS ➤

Tie an exercise band loosely just above your knees. Lie on your back with your arms down at your sides, and extend both legs straight up directly above your hips; your feet should be spread wide enough that the band is taut. Slowly open your legs as far as you can. Pause when the tension becomes too great to pull any farther, then slowly close back to the starting position.

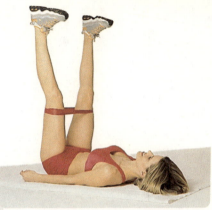

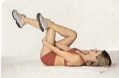

◄ **Follow with a Lying Figure-Four Stretch**
Lying faceup, cross your right ankle over your left knee, and pull your left leg (from behind the thigh) toward your chest. Switch legs.

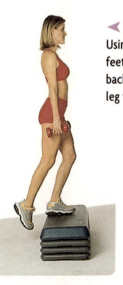

◄ **ADVANCED STEP-UP**

Using an aerobic step or regular step and holding dumbbells, start with both feet on the step. Keeping your left foot planted on the step, step off the back with your right foot. Before touching the floor, press up with your left leg to bring the right one up again. Repeat for one set, then switch legs.

➤ **Follow with a Lying Glute Stretch**
Lying faceup with legs extended, alternately pull each knee (grasping behind the thigh) toward your chest.

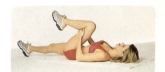

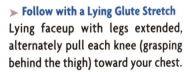

CHAPTER 5

Upper-Body Beautiful

Arm yourself for sleeveless styles with these torso-toning moves

Just a few years ago, women were dumbbell-phobic when it came to their upper bodies. Afraid that they'd get "muscles like a man," they steered clear of biceps curls and chest presses. Now, thanks to the sexy shoulders on celebs such as Halle Berry and Madonna, women see that a firm, toned upper body is definitely something to strive for. Fortunately, this problem spot is also a pretty quick fix. Since you have proportionately less fat on your arms than you do on your legs, and it's less "stubborn" (meaning that your hormones don't try to hang onto arm fat for famine protection), your arms respond more quickly

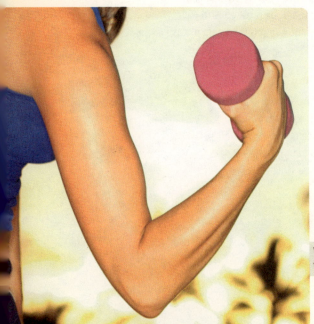

Wave goodbye to flabby arms.

to exercise, and you'll see results sooner. You'll also feel stronger.

Upper-body exercises also strengthen your spine, which can help prevent osteoporosis and protect you from developing a hunchback in your later years.

The following exercises will help firm and tone all of your upper-body muscles. For the most benefits, perform two or three sets of 8 to 12 reps of each of the following exercises. Repeat the exercises two or three times a week, but not on consecutive days.

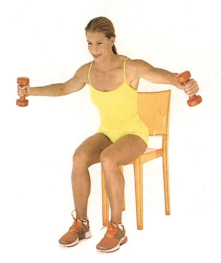

BACK FLY
MAJOR MUSCLES WORKED: **upper back**

Sit in a chair with your feet flat on the floor and about hip-width apart. Hold a dumbbell in each hand so the weights are at chest level and about 12 inches from your body. Your palms should be facing each other and your elbows slightly bent as if you were holding a beach ball. Bend forward from the hips about 3 to 5 inches. Keeping your back straight, squeeze your shoulder blades together, and pull your elbows back as far as comfortably possible. Pause, then return to the starting position. Repeat for 60 seconds.

CHEST PRESS
MAJOR MUSCLES WORKED: **chest and triceps**

Lying on the floor or a weight bench, hold dumbbells end to end just above chest height; your elbows should be pointing out. Press the dumbbells up, extending your arms. Hold, then lower.

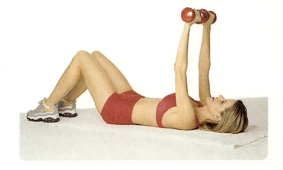

PUSH-UP
MAJOR MUSCLES WORKED: **chest, triceps, and back**

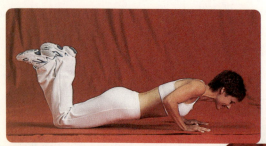

[1]

Start on your hands and knees, hands in line with your shoulders. Your hips should be extended so that your body forms a straight line from head to knees. Cross your ankles in the air. Push yourself up, then return to the starting position. Repeat. To make the move more challenging, extend your legs so you're balancing on your toes instead of your knees. (This is also a great on-the-go exercise.)

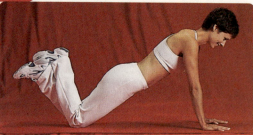

[2]

TURN UP THE BURN!

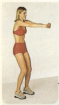

Stretch your workout rewards

Research shows that stretching after you strength train helps boost your benefits. Weave these three stretches into your upper-body routine for even greater results. Hold each for 15 seconds.

◄ **UPPER BACK STRETCH:** Extend both arms in front of you, and lace your fingertips together. As you press your palms away from you, round your back.

BENDING CHEST STRETCH: Place your hands on a chair or tabletop, and bend from the hips. Slowly drop your head between your arms so that your torso is parallel to the floor. ──────►

◄ **SHOULDER STRETCH:** Grasp your right elbow with your left hand, and gently pull your right arm across your chest. Keep your shoulder down. Switch arms.

Upper-body exercises strengthen your spine, which can help prevent osteoporosis and protect you from developing a hunchback in your later years.

ONE-ARM ROW
MAJOR MUSCLES WORKED: **back**

Put your left knee and left hand on a bench or chair, keeping your back flat. Hold a weight in your right hand with your right arm straight and the weight hanging toward the floor, parallel to the bench. Raise the weight, keeping it close to your body, until it's even with your waist; your elbow should be pointed toward the ceiling.

[1]

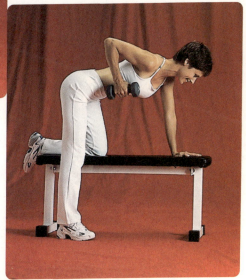

[2]

MILITARY PRESS
MAJOR MUSCLES WORKED: **shoulders**

While sitting on a bench or chair, hold a dumbbell in each hand. Start with the weights at shoulder height; your palms should be facing forward. Raise the weights above your head without bringing them together or locking your elbows, then bring them back down to your shoulders.

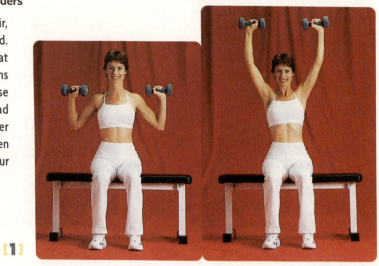

[1]

[2]

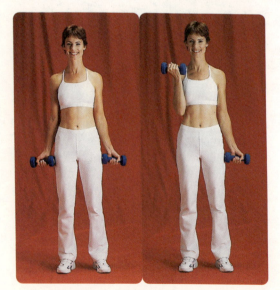

[1]

BICEPS CURL
MAJOR MUSCLES WORKED: **biceps**

Standing straight, hold a weight in each hand, palms facing forward. Keeping your elbow close to your body, bend your right arm, and lift the weight toward your shoulder. Return to the starting position, then repeat with your left arm.

[2]

TRICEPS EXTENSION
MAJOR MUSCLES WORKED: **triceps**

Sit on a bench or chair while holding a dumbbell in your left hand, palm facing in. Bend your arm, and raise it over your shoulder; your elbow will be pointing toward the ceiling, and the weight will be behind your head. Hold your left elbow steady with your right hand, and raise the weight until your arm is straight. Return to the starting position.

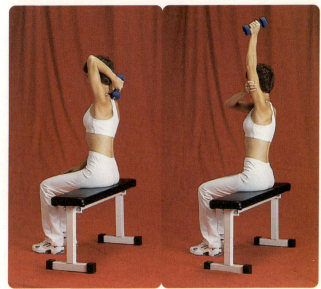

[1] [2]

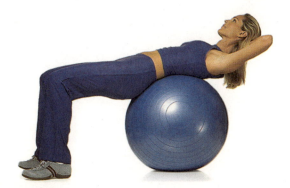

BALL CRUNCH
MAJOR MUSCLES WORKED: **abs**

Lie on your back on an exercise ball with your hands behind your head. Using your abs, raise your head and shoulders, and crunch your rib cage toward your pelvis. Pause, then slowly lower.

cardio blast!

40 **5 Steps to Cardio Success**
Turn on your fat burners with these workout tips

47 **Personalize Your Cardio Plan**
Discover the workouts that are perfect
for your personality and lifestyle

51 **Blast Fat to the Max!**
Kick your body-toning plan into high gear
with these fat-burning exercises

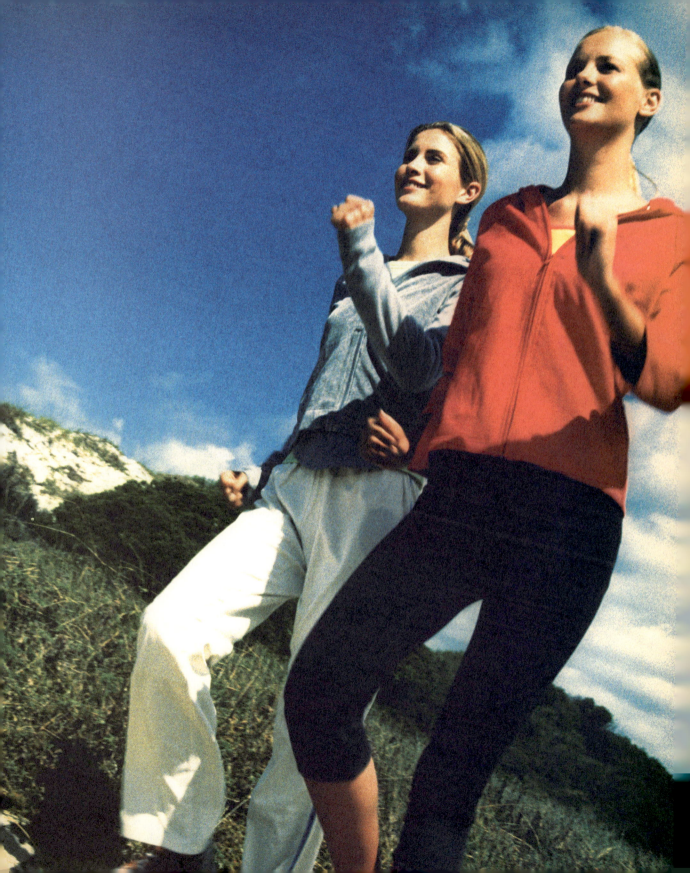

5 Steps to Cardio Success

Turn on your fat burners with these workout tips

If you take home only one message, make it this one: Moving your body through regular physical activity is the most important thing you can do for your health. It's more important than quitting smoking and more important than losing weight (though regular exercise can help you do both). Studies show that being sedentary is the biggest health risk of all. Getting regular cardiovascular exercise (that means 30 to 60 minutes) most days fights almost every ailment you can mention—plus, it fights fat! Here's just a sampling of the specific benefits regular exercisers enjoy.

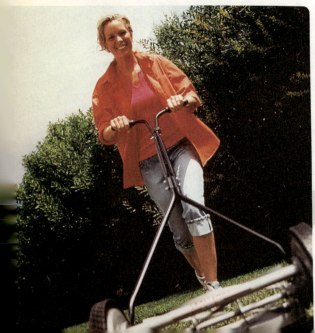

Get a gym-toned body in your own backyard.

• **A stronger, healthier heart.** Aerobic exercise makes the heart work harder, which makes it stronger: It pumps more blood with each beat, which means that it beats less often. In other words, aerobic exercise lowers your resting heart rate. It can also result in lower blood pressure because the blood moves more easily through arteries and veins. It also lowers cholesterol and burns abdominal fat. The end result is a lower risk of heart attack and stroke.

• **Cancer protection.** A number of studies have shown that exercise protects against colon cancer. It may lower the risk of breast and ovarian cancers as well.

• **Healthy blood sugar.** Exercise helps the body secrete insulin, which can reduce the risk of diabetes.

• **Fewer sick days.** Regular activity boosts immunity and can prevent colds and other infectious diseases.

• **Stronger bones.** Exercise strengthens your skeleton. Older women who are active suffer fewer bone fractures than women who don't exercise.

• **Revved-up metabolism.** Working out burns fat and builds muscle. It may also lower levels of leptin, a hormone that seems to contribute to weight gain. Studies show that the equivalent of just 3 hours a week of jogging can drop leptin levels by 10%.

• **Break bad habits.** In a study of 280 women, researchers at Brown University found that those who quit smoking and started exercising were twice as likely to stay smoke-free and gained half as much weight as women who quit without exercising.

• **Longer life.** A study of 14,000 people showed that moderate levels of physical fitness increased life span. In fact, walking as little as 2 miles daily could potentially add years to your life.

TURN UP THE BURN!

Make every move count

Every 15 minutes of exercise you do adds up to measurable results. Check out the calorie-burn chart below to see how your favorite activities stack up (based on a 140-lb woman who exercises for 15 minutes).

140 CALORIES
Mountain biking, hiking a moderate-to-difficult grade, snowshoeing in soft snow, running a 10-minute mile, running up stairs, doing karate or tae kwon do, kickboxing, jumping rope, swimming vigorously, using a stairclimber or ski machine

120 TO 139 CALORIES
Running a 12-minute mile, singles tennis, volleyball on the beach, downhill skiing, rock climbing, swimming laps, water jogging, having a snowball fight

95 TO 119 CALORIES
Backpacking, doubles tennis, racewalking, briskly walking uphill, jazz and modern dance, basketball, racquetball, soccer, high-impact aerobics, using a stationary rower, bicycling at a moderate pace, ice skating, sledding, shoveling snow

70 TO 94 CALORIES
Golf (carrying your clubs), downhill skiing on beginners' slopes, gardening, calisthenics, step aerobics, walking at a brisk pace, dancing (country, polka, or disco), playing tag, washing the car, using a snowblower, kayaking, mowing the lawn with a push mower

40 TO 69 CALORIES
Lawn and lane bowling, badminton, croquet, dancing (cha-cha or swing), tai chi, golf (using a cart), mowing the lawn on a riding mower, raking leaves, playing catch or Frisbee, walking the dog

Research has shown that women who exercise may have less menstrual discomfort. They're less anxious and depressed. They're more energetic. They have less back pain and more self-confidence. They even sleep better.

• **Improved well-being—today.** It's clear that exercise can improve the long-term quality (and quantity) of your life. But what will it do for you right now? Research has shown that women who exercise may have less menstrual discomfort. They're less anxious and depressed. They're more energetic. They have less back pain and more self-confidence. They even sleep better.

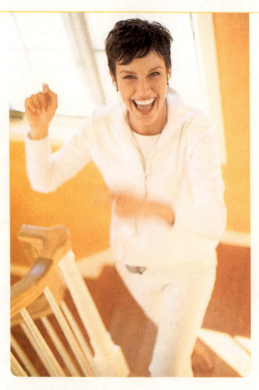

Getting in the Groove—
5 Steps to Success

So you *know* cardio is good for you. But maybe like 60% of Americans (more women than men), you still aren't getting regular physical activity. Or maybe you're a regular cardio junkie, but you've been doing the same old routine so long that it's no longer working the way it used to. Either way, you can benefit by following these time-tested tips for lasting cardio success. Ready? Get started!

STEP 1: Take the "Work" Out of Workout

The problem with formal exercise is that it can easily feel like one more responsibility in an already hectic day. But it shouldn't be like that. Exercise is any physical activity that you enjoy. Indulge some of the activities that are similar to what you enjoyed as a kid. Used to climb trees? Try rock climbing in the wild or on the "rock wall" at a local health club. Are you a dancer? Try one of the dance-oriented aerobics classes such as funk, swing, or salsa. Don't waste time doing something you don't enjoy very much. For years, women felt that they had to run in order to be aerobically fit. But a lot of them hated running, and naturally they didn't do it for very long. You have to do something that you like doing. It could be tennis. Bicycling. Climbing on the stairclimber. Or even line dancing.

STEP 2: Be Opportunistic

Look for exercise opportunities. Sure, running, biking, swimming, or other vigorous forms of exercise are great for physical fitness. But anything that gets your body moving counts, and the more the better! It can be walking the dog. Planting flowers. Raking leaves. Even cleaning the house can give you a decent workout if you move quickly and you do it for at least 30 minutes. "There are many ways to sneak in exercise," says Martha Coopersmith, owner of the Bodysmith Company in New York City. "We all have to go places, so park a couple of blocks away, and walk the rest. Take the stairs instead of the elevator. Or pace while you talk on the phone." Likewise, look for ways to eke a little more out of your regular workouts when you have the time and energy. Try to walk 10 more minutes than you usually do. Do one extra push-up. Lift the weights two more times.

Don't believe all those little motions add up to big exercise benefits? Consider this: Researchers have found that the laborsaving inventions of the past 25 years—everything from computers to remote controls—have shaved an average of 800 calories of daily activity from our lives. That's more than a pound a week! Any little thing you can do to burn a few more calories during the day will help.

STEP 3: Pump Up the Intensity

When you've been doing the same exercises for a while, you'll find that they get easier. This is because your body has adapted to the workload and is no longer feeling the strain. This is satisfying, in a way, because it means that you've made progress. But it also means that you won't progress further until you push your body a little harder.

To keep your workouts at maximum pitch, increase the intensity. In other words, lift more weight, run faster, and generally exercise harder two or three times a week. The boost in intensity can have substantial health and fitness benefits. One study found that people who regularly pushed their workouts to the limit had higher levels of high-density lipoprotein (HDL, the good cholesterol) than those who exercised at lower intensities.

There are a number of ways to boost the intensity of your workouts.

• **Go longer.** Suppose you're currently exercising for 30 minutes. To increase the intensity, kick it up to 35 minutes. Keep it at that level for a few weeks, then add another 5 minutes, then another. Exercising hard for 45 minutes will quickly add up to impressive fitness gains.

• **Add intervals.** Instead of going all out all the time—or, conversely, coasting along at a comfortable pace—shake things up with interval training. For example, exercise at a moderate pace for 4 minutes, then switch to high intensity for 4 minutes. Interval training will keep your body challenged without exhausting your muscles and lungs, says Wayne Westcott, PhD, fitness research director at the South Shore YMCA in Quincy, MA, and author of 15 books on strength training.

• **Add a new exercise.** Remember the strain you felt when you first started exercising? It's good to repeat the experience periodically because it puts a beneficial load on your whole body. As you challenge different muscles, your heart and lungs will work harder, and that's the cornerstone of boosting overall fitness.

• **Tune it up.** Sure, it's a good way to make the time go quickly, but music—as long as it has a fast tempo—also promotes impressive fitness gains.

In one study, 24 people cycled to music. The intensity of their cycling increased when they listened to music with a fast beat. The study's authors think that with the increase in the music's tempo, the participants were distracted from a preoccupation with how tired they felt.

STEP 4: Follow Your Heart Rate

You can exercise longer and burn more fat if you're in your target heart rate zone: not too easy, not too hard.

"One reason people quit exercising is that they push themselves too hard and feel fatigued or get injured," says Ed Burke, PhD, author of *Precision Heart Rate Training* (Human Kinetics, 1998). Likewise, some fail to see results because they never work hard enough. Tracking how many beats per minute (bpm) your heart pumps during exercise helps you adjust your workouts to maximize benefits.

To get your target heart rate zone, subtract your age from 220. That's your maximum heart rate (MHR). For best results, exercise within 60 to 80% of your MHR. If you're age 40, your MHR is 180 bpm (220 - 40), and your target range is 108 to 144 bpm (180 x .60; 180 x .80). This is just a

Listen to Your Heart
Pick the monitor that meets your needs

Monitoring your exercise heart rate can be motivational and help you burn fat faster. The best way to measure heart rate is with a heart rate monitor, a device (usually with a chest strap) that sends your heart rate signal to a monitor you wear on your wrist. Most also have special features such as stopwatches and alarms. Here's our review of some popular models.

HEARTALKER ($80)
Pros: talks you through your workout; easy to use; choose your coach: Denise Austin, Kathy Smith, or a male voice; no need for glasses to read a monitor
Cons: earpieces can be cumbersome; chest piece lost contact frequently; no visual cues
Ideal for a(n): exerciser who wants a no-brainer workout
For more info: (800) 915-5566; www.heartalker.com

POLAR A3 ($90)
Pros: simple to use and program; bold display; available in basic to multifeature models
Cons: transmission sometimes cuts out while running on treadmills
Ideal for a(n): exerciser who wants bare-bones, consistent heart rate info
For more info: (800) 227-1314; in Canada, toll-free (888) 918-5043; www.polarusa.com

rough estimate. Always consider how you feel too.

Check your heart rate by taking your pulse at your wrist or neck. For an easier, more accurate reading, try a heart rate monitor. (See "Listen to Your Heart" on p. 44.)

Knowing your heart rate may also save your life someday. In a 6-year study of more than 2,400 people, cardiologists at the Cleveland Clinic in Ohio found that "heart rate recovery," how quickly your heart rate drops after exercise, is an important predictor of heart attack risk. Those who had slow recovery rates were four times as likely to die as people with normal recovery rates. "About a

minute after a moderately hard workout such as a jog, your heart rate should drop by at least 12 beats," says lead researcher Michael Lauer, MD. If it stays high, see your doctor.

STEP 5: Mix It Up!

While exercise consistency is important, infusing variety into our daily routine increases our strength and aerobic capacities faster than doing the exact same thing every day, with less likelihood of dropping out or injuring ourselves. It's also a whole lot more fun. To understand the magic of cross-training, it helps to understand the

TIMEX IRONMAN ($125)
Pros: great transmission (reading never cut out); offers many special sports features
Cons: large, uncomfortable chest strap; too complex for basic exercisers
Ideal for a(n): competitive exerciser who wants to track training progress
For more info: (800) 367-8463; www.timex.com

MIO ($130)
Pros: no chest strap; includes calorie-tracking feature
Cons: didn't work for every tester; can't use while running or biking
Ideal for a(n): walker who is uncomfortable with chest straps
For more info: toll-free (877) 566-4636; www.gophysical.com

FITSENSE FS-1 ($239)
Pros: includes a pedometer to give walking/running pace
Cons: hard-to-read display; complicated to program
Ideal for a(n): die-hard walker or gadget junkie
For more info: (800) 419-3667; www.fitsense.com

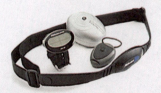

Begin and end wisely

Make your cardio routines safer and more enjoyable by giving yourself 5 to 10 minutes to warm up and 5 to 10 minutes to cool down and stretch.

metabolism of muscle building. When you challenge a muscle by bench-pressing a weight or pedaling a bicycle, it responds by first breaking down, then (with rest) building back up stronger and more solid. Those new and improved muscle fibers burn more calories and help you shed unwanted fat. As long as you keep riding farther or faster or lifting more weight, those muscles will continue to break down, build up, get stronger, and burn fat.

Problem is that you can ride only so far or bench-press only so much weight. When you reach the point where you're going through the same motions at the same intensity, your muscles adapt and stop getting stronger, so you burn fewer calories. How long it takes to reach this point depends on your current fitness level, but fitness scientists believe that muscles begin to adapt to repetitive movements in just 2 to 4 weeks. All it takes is little changes to keep your body guessing—and working.

Always aim for a balanced blend of fitness activities. If you're spinning on Mondays, make it a point to try in-line skating on Wednesdays to challenge your leg muscles in a completely different way. Mix high-intensity activities such as kickboxing with low-intensity exercise such as yoga. The more muscles you can work from different angles in different ways, the more effective your exercise routine will be.

CHAPTER 7

Personalize Your Cardio Plan

Discover the workouts that are perfect for your personality and lifestyle

Choose activities that mesh well with who you are and what you like to do, and you'll be more likely to stick to them. The following quiz will help you identify activities you will enjoy and keep enjoying, based on your personality, workout goals, and schedule. Take each section of the quiz, and combine the results of the three parts to get your total fitness personality. Then read "Blast Fat to the Max!" on p. 51 to learn more about activities that are perfect for your personality.

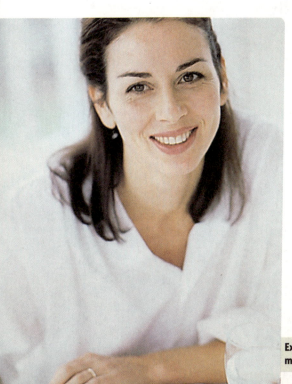

Exercise should make you smile.

PART 1: What Makes You Tick?

1. As a kid, the activities I liked best were:

a) gymnastics, cheerleading, jumping rope, or dance classes

b) playing outside: building forts or lemonade stands, climbing trees, exploring the woods, etc.

c) competitive sports

d) playing with dolls, reading, coloring, or art projects

e) parties; playing with my friends

2. My favorite hobbies today are:

a) anything new and challenging

b) outside activities: gardening, walking the dog, watching the stars, etc.

c) tennis, card or board games, team and/or spectator sports

d) reading, movies, needle crafts, painting, or anything that provides an escape

e) group activities with friends: anything from a walking club or joining a book group to just talking

3. I get motivated to exercise if:

a) I get a new exercise video or piece of equipment, or I try a totally new class

b) I get a new piece of exercise equipment I can use outside, I discover a new walking or jogging path, or the weather is nice

c) I'm presented with some competition

d) I find an exercise that I really get into to the point that I forget my surroundings

e) I exercise in a group

4. I prefer to exercise:

a) indoors, in a gym or at home

b) outdoors

c) wherever there's competition

d) wherever I'm not the center of attention

e) in a gym or fitness center

INTERPRETING YOUR SCORE FOR PART 1

MOSTLY A'S OR A MIXTURE OF LETTERS: **The Learner.** You're always trying something new. You are most likely an "associative exerciser," meaning you focus on the way your body moves and feels when you exercise. Choose activities that help you explore new moves. Try aerobics classes, African dance, Pilates, Tae-Bo, tai chi, inline skating, jumping rope, fencing, or BOSU (aerobics on a springy stability dome).

MOSTLY B'S: **Outdoors Woman.** Fresh air is your energizer. So why not include nature in your exercise routine? Try hiking, biking, nature walking, gardening, lap swimming, or cross-country skiing. If you have a piece of home exer-

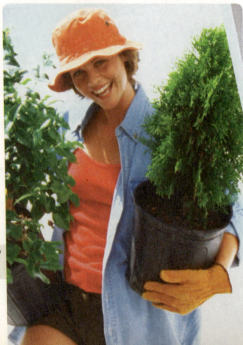

Love the outdoors? Get fresh-air fit!

cise equipment you love, drag it out to the patio on a nice day. Or do yoga on your back porch.

MOSTLY C'S: **Competitor.** You naturally like one-on-one, competitive types of activities. Try fencing, cardio kickboxing, Tae-Bo, tai chi, or spinning classes. If you excelled in or enjoyed a sport when you were younger, take it up again.

MOSTLY D'S: **Timid Gal.** You're a "disassociative exerciser," meaning you fantasize or think of events in your life when you exercise, rather than the exercise itself. You will like mind/body activities such as yoga and Pilates. Also try nature walking or hiking as well as some group classes such as spinning, step aerobics, Tae-Bo, tai chi, and water aerobics.

MOSTLY E'S: **Social Butterfly.** As a people person, you tend to prefer the gym to exercising in your living room. Try aerobics classes, kickboxing, yoga, spinning classes, step aerobics, water aerobics, Tae-Bo, and tai chi classes. For weight lifting, find a buddy or two, and do circuit training.

PART 2: Workout Style & Goals

5. My primary exercise goal is:

    a) to lose weight/tone up

    b) to relax and/or relieve stress

    c) to have fun

    d) depends on how I feel

6. I prefer:

    a) a lot of structure in my workout

    b) some structure, but not too much

    c) no structure

    d) depends on my mood

7. I prefer to exercise:

    a) alone

    b) with one other person

    c) in a group

    d) depends on my mood

INTERPRETING YOUR SCORE FOR PART 2

MOSTLY A'S: **Gung-ho Exerciser.** You exercise to tone up, period. No messing around. You'll benefit most from doing a specific activity, such as cycling, aerobics, using elliptical machines, treadmills, stairclimbers, etc. at a moderate intensity. For optimal weight loss, perform 30 minutes of aerobic-based exercise daily, and combine this with three sessions of weight training a week.

MOSTLY B'S: **Leisurely Exerciser.** Your main exercise objectives are to relax and de-stress. To relax, try yoga. Also, studies have shown a direct relationship between physical activity and stress reduction. Hop on the treadmill, or head outside and walk for 5 minutes, run slowly for 30 seconds, then run fast for 30 seconds, repeating this sequence for about 30 minutes.

MOSTLY C'S: **Fun-Loving Exerciser.** Fifty straight minutes on the treadmill is not your bag. Grab your inline skates, and circle the neighborhood. Put on your favorite music CD, and dance around the living room. Make your weight routine more amusing by doing circuit weight training (moving from one exercise to the next with minimal rest).

MOSTLY D'S: **Flexible Exerciser.** Exercise turns you on, but routine doesn't. You'd rather fly by the seat of your gym shorts, which is fine. To add variety, use the elliptical machine one day, the treadmill the next, and the cross-country skiing machine the next.

PART 3: Lifestyle/Schedule

8. I have the most energy:

a) in the morning

b) in the middle of the day

c) in the evening or at night

d) my energy level fluctuates

9. I have the most time:

a) in the morning

b) in the middle of the day

c) in the evening

d) depends on the day

10. I'm most likely to:

a) go to bed early and get up early

b) go to bed and get up at the same time every day, but not particularly early or late

c) go to bed late and get up late

d) depends on the day

INTERPRETING YOUR SCORE FOR PART 3

MOSTLY A'S: **Morning Dove.** You like to get chores out of the way as soon as you get up because that's when you have the most energy. Whether you go to the gym before you start your day or you head outside for a dawn walk, you'll have an extra edge over those who hit the snooze button a few more times.

MOSTLY B'S: **Midday Duck.** You'd rather plop down on an exercise bike than in front of a sandwich when noon rolls around. Fine. Whether you're at home or work, exercise is a great way to break up your day.

MOSTLY C'S: **Night Owl.** You haven't seen a sunrise since that all-night party in 1974. If you have more energy at night, exercise then. Just don't do it too close to bedtime, or you'll have trouble sleeping.

MOSTLY D'S OR AN EVEN MIXTURE OF LETTERS: **Flexible Bird.** The best time of day for you to exercise varies with your schedule. Just go with it.

Excerpted from Fit Not Fat at 40-Plus, *copyright 2002, Rodale Inc. To order, call (800) 848-4735, or visit www.rodalestore.com.*

CHAPTER 8

Blast Fat to the Max!

Kick your body-toning plan into high gear with these fat-burning exercises

If strength training is the best way to build muscle, cardio exercise is the best way to make those new muscles shine. Aerobic workouts are a great way to burn calories and melt away excess fat that's covering your newly toned muscles, leaving you looking shapely and lean.

To help you maximize your cardio time, here's a review of 12 types of aerobic exercise. Try a variety of activities to keep yourself motivated. Just take your pick, and you can get started today!

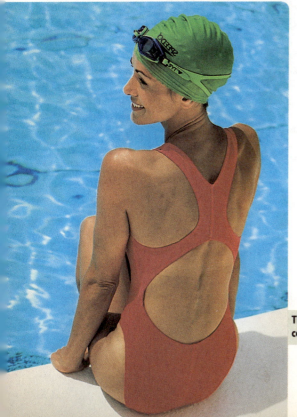

These moves will make you confident about your body.

Aerobics Classes and Videotapes

For weight loss, an aerobics workout can hardly be beat, says Laurie L. Tis, PhD, associate professor in the department of kinesiology and health at Georgia State University in Atlanta. And for muscle toning, aerobics also incorporates resistance exercises that add up to a sleek physique.

More than choreographed calisthenics, today's aerobics classes and videotapes challenge you to kickbox, jump rope, do tennis swings, and more, with background tunes ranging from reggae to urban funk. You can also choose from a variety of new high-energy classes such as rebounding and BOSU, which use trampolines and other bouncy props to give the class extra kick.

AEROBICS CLASSES AND VIDEOTAPES STATS

CALORIES BURNED*	BODY-SHAPING BONUS
228 per half hour	Tones abdominals, hips, thighs, buttocks, and (depending on type of aerobics performed) other major muscles

* Based on a 150-lb woman. If you weigh more, you'll burn more calories; if you weigh less, you'll burn fewer.

WORKOUTS

Beginner 10 to 20 minutes, 3 days a week; target heart rate 60 to 65% of maximum

Intermediate 20 to 30 minutes, 3 to 5 days a week; target heart rate 65 to 75% of maximum

Experienced Minimum 20 to 30 minutes, 3 to 5 days a week; target heart rate 75 to 90% of maximum

The best approach to exercise intensity is to work at your own pace, says Lauri Reimer, director of aerobic instructor training for the Aerobics and Fitness Association of America in Sherman Oaks, CA. "In a class, don't worry about keeping up with the people in the front row," she advises. Do 5 leg kicks instead of 10 if that's all you can handle right now. Jump, but skip the arm-reaching part of jumping jacks. Just keep moving. "The point is to do as much as you can, and aim for improvement over time," Reimer says.

For maximum weight loss, work out for 30 to 60 minutes at moderate intensity most days of the week.

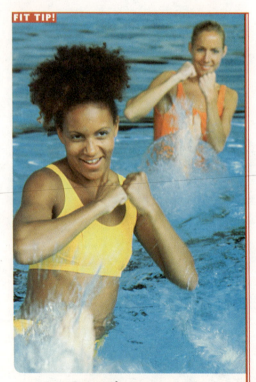

FIT TIP!

Get wet!
Aerobics can be done not only on a mat or exercise floor but also in a pool. You'll burn about 200 to 250 calories per half hour of water aerobics.

Bicycling

There's no better way to feel like a kid again than swinging your leg over a bicycle. Yet bicycling definitely isn't just for kids; it's also a great workout for adults. "If your knees, ankles, or hips bother you when you walk, then cycling might be a great, pain-free way to exercise and lose weight," says Edmund Burke, PhD, professor of exercise science at the University of Colorado in Colorado Springs and coauthor of *Fitness Cycling*. "Unlike walking or running, cycling isn't a weight bearing exercise. The bicycle, not your bones and joints, supports your weight."

BICYCLING STATS

CALORIES BURNED*	BODY-SHAPING BONUS
130–145 per half hour, depending on your speed and the terrain	Strengthens and tones all the muscles of your lower body, including your butt, thighs, and calves

* Based on a 150-lb woman. If you weigh more, you'll burn more calories; if you weigh less, you'll burn fewer.

WORKOUTS

Beginner Cycle nonstop for 20 minutes on flat terrain, two or three times a week for 3 to 4 weeks.

Intermediate Beginning on flat terrain, cycle fast for 20 to 30 minutes. Then include a couple of hills, or shift to a harder gear for 5 minutes at a time, without necessarily going fast. Do this three times a week until you work your way up to riding comfortably 60 minutes each time.

Experienced Extend one of your regularly scheduled rides, probably on the weekend, to at least 1½ to 2 times the time or distance of a weekday ride. Vary the speed and intensity as you ride: Climb hills, ride quickly for a few minutes, and use more intensity at other times.

When you first start to cycle, don't try to conquer hills or ride for a set amount of time, says Dr. Burke. Instead, choose flat terrain. "You want to feel successful each time you ride, so you look forward to getting on the bike again the next time," he says.

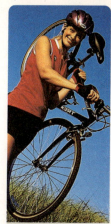

The perfect weight loss machine.

Elliptical Training

An elliptical trainer looks like a combination treadmill, cross-country ski machine, and stepping machine, and it combines the movements (and benefits) of hiking, cross-country skiing, and biking. Instead of your feet moving back and forth like a ski machine, an elliptical trainer forces them to move around in an oval (or elliptical) pattern.

Using the elliptical trainer doesn't create any impact, so it's easy on your joints. And it's versatile: You can use it to climb or glide. For your effort, you'll get a calorie-burning workout that pumps your heart like an all-out run without the stress and strain on the joints in your body.

ELLIPTICAL TRAINING STATS

CALORIES BURNED*	BODY-SHAPING BONUS
500–600 per hour	Tones muscles of the entire lower body and burns fat

* Based on a 150-lb woman. If you weigh more, you'll burn more calories; if you weigh less, you'll burn fewer.

WORKOUTS

Beginner Two or three times a week for 10 to 20 minutes at a time in a slow rhythm

Intermediate Two or three times a week for at least 20 minutes, using a preprogrammed workout that doesn't include intervals

Experienced Two or three times a week for 20 to 60 minutes of interval training, either preprogrammed or self-directed

"At first, start off with 10 minutes of elliptical training at a low intensity," says J. Zack Barksdale, an exercise physiologist at The Cooper Aerobics Center in Dallas. "Do this twice a week for 1 week, then begin to change the workouts. To do this, increase something every week, but don't increase two things at once. For example, in the second week you could increase the number of times you exercise from two to three. Then in the third week, you might increase your intensity."

Hiking

If you want to jazz up your walking routine, take to the trails. "Hiking is like walking, with one major difference: It takes you to new and exciting terrain," says Don Heil, PhD, assistant professor of exercise physiology at Montana State University in Bozeman.

HIKING STATS

CALORIES BURNED*	BODY-SHAPING BONUS
250 per half hour	Tones the legs and butt; also increases aerobic endurance

* Based on a 150-lb woman. If you weigh more, you'll burn more calories; if you weigh less, you'll burn fewer.

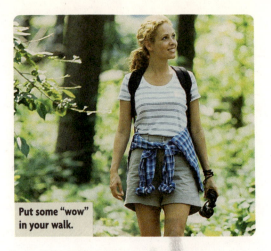
Put some "wow" in your walk.

WORKOUTS

Beginner 20 to 30 minutes of hiking on a trail or a beach three times a week

Intermediate 40 minutes of hiking 5 or 6 days a week, plus a long hike (60 minutes) up and over a mountain on Saturday

Experienced Longer hikes (2 to 4 hours) on rockier terrain; for highly experienced hikers, adventures that last for more than 4 hours

"Distance, terrain, and weather conditions can make a hike challenging," says Dr. Heil. Few hikers worry about speed. "Hiking isn't a race," he says. "If anything, it's leisurely. Even when the terrain is challenging, you're taking time to notice just how beautiful nature is."

Hiking a mile on a trail isn't the same as walking a mile on flat ground. Distances can be deceiving. So pay attention to guidebook estimates of how long a trail is, the elevation gained, and how much time it takes to hike.

Stay Injury-Free
Surefire steps for preventing strains and pains

Nothing will get you off your path to fitness and firmness faster than an injury. You can avoid common sports injuries with a few simple steps, says Nicholas DiNubile, MD, an orthopedic surgeon in Havertown, PA.

START WARM AND LIMBER. Like taffy, muscles are brittle when cold and pliable when warm. Exercise lightly at first, and stretch a little.

ADD VARIETY. Alternate activities to avoid overusing particular body parts.

TAKE LESSONS. Many overuse injuries, such as tennis elbow, stem from poor technique or improperly fitted equipment.

ALTERNATE INTENSITY. If you worked out hard yesterday, go easier today. Give your body 1 day of rest a week.

LISTEN TO YOUR ACHES. If you have pain, especially in your joints, see a sports medicine specialist.

PLAY YOUR SPORT SENSIBLY. Every sport requires special precautions. Here's what the American Academy of Orthopaedic Surgeons recommends.

➤ **Basketball:** Wear snug, nonskid basketball shoes as well as ankle supports.
➤ **Bicycling:** Choose a helmet in the smallest size that's comfortable. Then wear it. Older adults wear helmets less frequently than kids—and die of head injuries twice as often as a result.
➤ **Golf:** Avoid tight waistbands that can pull on your lower back when you swing.
➤ **In-line skating:** Wear a helmet and protective joint pads. Master the skills of stopping and turning before you venture into busy areas or go near traffic.
➤ **Running, jogging:** Shoes lose 60% of their shock absorption after 250 to 500 miles and should be replaced.
➤ **Soccer:** Wear shin guards. Use synthetic, nonabsorbent balls; leather balls can get too heavy in damp conditions.
➤ **Softball, baseball:** Save your arm. Throw no more than 80 to 100 pitches per week (about 4 to 10 innings) or one game per week.
➤ **Tennis:** Avoid landing on the balls of your feet. When hitting overhead, don't arch your back.
➤ **Volleyball:** Use knee pads if you dive for balls. "Call" for the ball to avoid collisions.

Jogging and Treadmill Running

Jogging gives you more bang for your buck than walking, since it uses the same muscle groups but burns calories faster. "You can generally figure on burning 100 calories a mile," says Ellen Glickman-Weiss, PhD, associate professor of exercise physiology in the department of exercise, leisure, and sports at Kent State University in Ohio. "Walking 1 mile may take you 15 to 20 minutes; jogging will take you half as long. Both are tremendous for overall fitness benefits," she explains. Simply defined as running slowed down, jogging offers less risk of injury than full-out running while providing top-notch aerobic benefits.

JOGGING AND TREADMILL RUNNING STATS

CALORIES BURNED*	BODY-SHAPING BONUS
102 per mile	Firms the calves, thighs, butt, and, to a lesser extent, abs

Based on a 150-lb woman. If you weigh more, you'll burn more calories; if you weigh less, you'll burn fewer.

WORKOUTS

Beginner Alternate jogging and walking for 20 minutes a day, 3 to 5 days a week.

Intermediate Jog 40 minutes at least 4 or 5 days a week.

Experienced Jog for an hour up to five times a week, not to exceed 30 miles per week. Beyond 30 miles, there is really no extra benefit, and your risk of injury increases.

To be sure you're working hard enough (but not too hard), keep track of your heart rate as you jog. To determine your ideal maximum heart rate range—an intensity that's neither too easy nor too hard—subtract your age from 220. Multiply that number by 0.6; that's your lower-limit heart rate for exercise. Next, multiply the same number by 0.9; that's your upper limit.

Jumping Rope

For any busy woman, jumping rope is the ultimate calorie-burning exercise. It doesn't take a lot of time, it's high intensity (so you'll burn lots of calories fast), and it's inexpensive.

JUMPING ROPE STATS

CALORIES BURNED*	BODY-SHAPING BONUS
110–130 per 10-minute session	Firms up the butt and thigh muscles and develops the calf muscles

Based on a 150-lb woman. If you weigh more, you'll burn more calories; if you weigh less, you'll burn fewer.

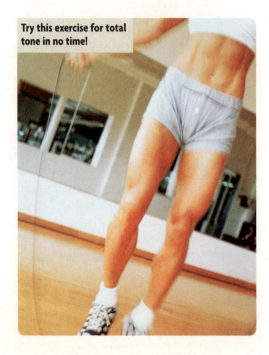

Try this exercise for total tone in no time!

Beginner Do 5 to 20 minutes of easy, two-footed jumping, paying attention to form. Start out with five 1-minute sessions between other interval activities. Work up to doing 1-minute jumping intervals for half the time. Do this combination three or four times a week.

Intermediate Do 20 to 40 minutes of two-footed jumping—or alternating between one-footed and two-footed jumping—three or four times a week. Jump for 2-minute intervals, broken up by 3 minutes of another activity, so you are jumping two-thirds of the time.

Experienced Alternate 3 minutes of jumping with 3 minutes of other activities for a total of 40 to 60 minutes.

When it comes to choosing an aerobic exercise, think of jumping rope as the polar opposite of walking. It takes about 23 minutes to burn 100 calories when you walk, whereas you'll easily burn more than 100 calories in just 15 minutes of jumping rope.

Once you get the general rhythm of jumping, try to extend your workout until you can jump for 2 to 3 minutes before taking a break.

Snowshoeing

When the temperature drops and the skies shade to gray, avoiding winter fat insulation can become a major mission. Now there's a cold-weather workout that can whip you into shape quicker than any of your favorite summer sports. It's snowshoeing, the fastest-growing winter sport among women. It's easy, safe, and invigorating, and it incinerates calories like a coal furnace in February.

The excitement over this activity is due to the miracles of modern technology. Snowshoes used to be huge, unwieldy wooden paddles awkwardly strapped to your feet, forcing you to walk like you just got off a horse. But today's shoes, made of synthetic materials, are lightweight, flexible, and contoured. In short, if you can walk, you can snowshoe. It's also pretty cheap. You can rent shoes from some retail stores and ski shops for about $10 a day, or you can buy your own pair for less than $100. All you need is some snow, and you're off!

SNOWSHOEING STATS

CALORIES BURNED*	BODY-SHAPING BONUS
272 per half hour; more if you're on hilly terrain or in deep snow	Blasts thighs, glutes, and calves; tones arms, back, and chest if you use ski poles

* Based on a 150-lb woman. If you weigh more, you'll burn more calories; if you weigh less, you'll burn fewer.

WORKOUTS

Beginner 45 to 60 minutes trekking across flat, not-too-deep, or broken-in snow

Intermediate 60 minutes trekking across rolling terrain; or snowshoeing through deep (10+ inches) or fresh snow

Experienced 60+ minutes of snowshoeing on challenging, hilly terrain; or snowshoeing through deep (10+ inches) or fresh snow

Although they're not a necessity, a pair of ski poles can greatly add to your snowshoeing enjoyment. They improve your balance, especially on the uphills and downhills. Your legs won't fatigue as fast with your arms helping out. And as a bonus, trekking with poles burns more calories and builds the muscles in your upper body.

Stationary Cycling

If you prefer an at-home workout that allows you to read or watch TV while you exercise, stationary cycling is a good choice. It's also a good alternative to outdoor activities when the weather is cold or wet. Yet another way to take advantage of stationary cycling is to use it as an "easy" workout once or twice a week, giving yourself a break from more intense aerobic activities you participate in.

STATIONARY CYCLING STATS

CALORIES BURNED*	BODY-SHAPING BONUS
130–330 per half hour	Tones your leg and glute muscles

* *Based on a 150-lb woman. If you weigh more, you'll burn more calories; if you weigh less, you'll burn fewer.*

WORKOUTS

Beginner Progressive intervals: Over a 22-minute period, intersperse slow-paced, low-intensity riding with short, higher-intensity spurts. Ride at a slow pace and low intensity for 5 minutes, then pedal for 30 seconds at higher intensity. Keep alternating, but end up with some slow pedaling to cool down.

Intermediate Pyramid workout: Ride for 10 minutes at high intensity, then follow with 2 minutes of low-intensity riding. Then do 8 minutes at a level of intensity that's even higher than the first 10 minutes, followed by another 2-minute, low-intensity interlude. Each increasingly harder interval should be 2 minutes shorter than the one before, but keep on increasing the intensity, and always insert a 2-minute interval to cool down. The whole routine should take about 40 minutes. Give yourself some slow pedaling at the end to finish off.

Experienced Hill training: If you want to test your maximum capacity, plan on riding for a certain amount of time (say, 40 minutes), and use progressively higher resistance throughout the ride. Increase the resistance every 3 to 4 minutes to increase the intensity of your workout. When you are halfway through the session, decrease the resistance at regular intervals over the same amount of time.

Stepping and Stairclimbing Machines

Stepping machines not only burn off overall fat, but they give definition to the muscles of your lower body, including the glutes, hamstrings, quadriceps (in your thighs), and gastrocnemius (in your calves). As the fat melts away, the long, lean muscles underneath are revealed.

Although the terms stepper and stairclimber are used interchangeably, they are two different machines. Steppers work only your lower body. You balance on the handlebars, pushing with one foot at a time alternately. Climbers work the whole body.

STEPPING AND STAIRCLIMBING MACHINES STATS

CALORIES BURNED*	BODY-SHAPING BONUS
250–350 calories per half hour	Tones butt, thighs, hips, and calves

* *Based on a 150-lb woman. If you weigh more, you'll burn more calories; if you weigh less, you'll burn fewer.*

WORKOUTS

Beginner Do 5 minutes at the lowest level you feel comfortable with, every day if possible. Work your way up to 20 minutes at this intensity.

Intermediate Once you can do 20 minutes of exercise every day, cut down on frequency, but increase intensity. Exercise for 2 days on and 1 day off, raising the intensity level every few workouts.

Get fit in just 12 minutes a day

Studies show that just several minutes of stairclimbing each day can help you lose weight, improve fitness, and reduce cardiovascular disease risk in only a few weeks.

In a British study, 12 sedentary women climbed a 200-step staircase, progressing from once a day to six times a day. (They took the elevator down.) Each ascent took about 2 minutes, so by the end of the study, the women were exercising only 12 minutes a day. In less than 2 months, they raised their fitness level and reduced their cholesterol levels enough to cut their risk of cardiovascular disease by 33%!

Aim for 20 minutes, three or four times a week.

Experienced Alternate between high and moderate intensity: For every minute of high-intensity exercise, do 2 minutes of moderate-intensity work. Continue for 20 minutes, three or four times a week.

Don't try to go all out when you first mount a stepping machine, say experts. "If you start small and go slow, you'll eventually be able to light up the display monitor on your machine for relatively long, intense workouts," says Cedric X. Bryant, PhD, senior vice president of research and development/sports medicine at the Stair-Master Corporation in Kirkland, WA. "The key is to begin with short workouts that are within your capabilities."

Swimming

Swimming may be the perfect way for a woman who needs to lose a few pounds to begin an exercise program, because extra fat helps keep you buoyant, making it easier to swim better and faster.

"Swimming isn't weight bearing; it doesn't subject your joints and bones to a lot of added impact," says Jane Katz, EdD, professor of health and physical education at the John Jay College of Criminal Justice of City University of New York and author of *The All-American Aquatic Handbook and Swimming for Total Fitness*. "You're expending a lot of energy, which burns calories, but you don't have to support the weight of your whole body while you do it."

SWIMMING STATS

CALORIES BURNED*	BODY-SHAPING BONUS
249–351 per half hour, depending on what stroke you do and how fast	Great calorie burner; tones the legs, hips, torso, arms, back, and chest

* Based on a 150-lb woman. If you weigh more, you'll burn more calories; if you weigh less, you'll burn fewer.

WORKOUTS

Beginner Swim freestyle laps for a total of 100 to 300 yards every other day or at least three times a week for 1 to 2 months. If you have to stop in between laps at first, that's okay. Work up to swimming nonstop for 10 minutes. If you use fins, you'll burn more calories.

Intermediate Swim 350 to 550 yards in about 15 minutes without stopping, at least three times a week for 2 months.

Experienced Swim 600 to 880 yards at a time without stopping, three times a week. Mix and match your strokes if you want. This should take about 30 minutes.

Get Fit in Your Living Room

Here's a guide to the best home equipment money can buy

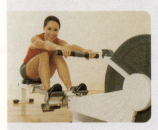

Nothing beats home fitness equipment when you just can't get to the gym. But buying the right machine is critical. Too often, that product that looked so great in the infomercial doesn't perform as promised and ends up as an expensive clothes hanger.

Avoid this by choosing equipment that you could see yourself using at least 3 days a week. To help you decide, here's everything you need to know about the most popular home equipment.

Elliptical

Pros: Easy on joints; low risk of injury; lots of programs (walk, hike, cross-country ski), so you train more muscles

Cons: Takes some getting used to; requires good coordination

It's a good choice for you if you... have joint problems; want to cross-train; are rehabbing an injury

Size: *(1 to 5 scale, with 1 being the smallest)*: **5**

Cost of a good model: $1,000–$3,000

Ease of use *(1 to 5 scale, with 1 being the easiest)*: **3**—Not a natural motion, but you can go at a slow pace, and it's low impact.

Miscellaneous: Most home versions have arm handles for an upper-body workout.

Rower

Pros: Works the upper and lower body at the same time; can build some muscle strength and endurance

Cons: May aggravate back problems; awkward to get off and on; not weight bearing, so bones don't benefit as much

It's a good choice for you if you... are fit; enjoy rowing; want a challenge

Size: *(1 to 5 scale, with 1 being the smallest)*: **5**

Cost of a good model: $300–$1,000

Ease of use *(1 to 5 scale, with 1 being the easiest)*: **5**—Not a natural motion, and it's a tough all-body workout.

Miscellaneous: Choose a model with air or water resistance.

Stairclimber

Pros: Easy to read on it; good for legs, buttocks, and bones (because it's weight bearing)

Cons: Bad for knee or ankle problems; potential for repetitive use injuries

It's a good choice for you if you... are fit; looking for a big calorie burner; want to do something else while exercising

Size: *(1 to 5 scale, with 1 being the smallest)*: **2**

Cost of a good model: $500–$2,000

Ease of use *(1 to 5 scale, with 1 being the easiest)*: **4**—A natural motion, but a tough workout because you're lifting your body weight.

Miscellaneous: Don't lean on the arm rails; take steps that are about 8 inches high; hydraulic models are prone to problems.

Stationary Bike

Pros: Easiest machine to multitask on (read, make phone calls, etc.)

Cons: Boring (all you do is pedal); not weight bearing, so no help for bones

It's a good choice for you if you... are very heavy; are unfit; have joint, balance, or dizziness problems

Size: *(1 to 5 scale, with 1 being the smallest)*: **1** (recumbent models take up more room)

Cost of a good model: $300–$500

Ease of use *(1 to 5 scale, with 1 being the easiest)*: **2**—Most people know how to pedal, and you get to sit.

Miscellaneous: Recumbent styles are easier than uprights; padded shorts are strongly recommended.

Treadmill

Pros: Lots of variety (walk, run, hills); weight bearing, so good for bones and calorie burning

Cons: See "size" and "cost" categories.

It's a good choice for you if you... can walk, regardless of your fitness level

Size: *(1 to 5 scale, with 1 being the smallest)*: **3**—Choose a folding model if you don't have a lot of room.

Cost of a good model: $500–$3,000

Ease of use *(1 to 5 scale, with 1 being the easiest)*: **1**—It's the most natural motion.

Miscellaneous: Choose a higher-quality model if you plan to run on it; make sure the size of the belt suits your body size.

Sources: Gregory Florez, spokesperson for the American Council on Exercise; John Porcari, PhD, professor in the department of exercise and sports science, University of Wisconsin-LaCrosse; Wayne Westcott, PhD, Prevention advisor and fitness research director at the South Shore YMCA in Quincy, MA.

Swimming *(continued)*

"This beginner program is designed for someone who knows how to swim but hasn't been doing laps regularly," says Dr. Katz. "Wearing swim fins, you'll start out swimming slowly and gradually increase your speed over the course of a few months." To warm up, walk in the shallow part of the pool, or tread water in place.

Tennis

Now here's a woman's sport. Chris Evert, Martina Navratilova, Jennifer Capriati, Serena and Venus Williams, Martina Hingis—great players, all. You don't have to play like a pro, however, to develop a slammin' body. "When I look at the women who play tennis consistently at our club, they're all in pretty good shape," says Jim Coyne, director of tennis at the Claremont Resort in Berkeley, CA.

If you haven't played tennis since high school, or if you've never picked up a racket, you may want a few lessons to brush up on your technique. But either way, if you're looking for a fun way to work more exercise into your life, this centuries-old sport is definitely worth a try. (You don't even have to wear a teeny white skirt—unless you want to.)

TENNIS STATS

CALORIES BURNED*	BODY-SHAPING BONUS
237 per half hour of vigorous play	Tones and firms glutes, thighs, calves, and shoulders

* Based on a 150-lb woman. If you weigh more, you'll burn more calories; if you weigh less, you'll burn fewer.

WORKOUTS

Beginner Enjoy noncompetitive play for at least half an hour against someone of equal or greater ability than yourself.

Intermediate Play competitively for 45 minutes to an hour.

Experienced Engage in 60 to 90 minutes of vigorous, competitive play

Wearing the right shoes is important in tennis. Running shoes and cross-trainers don't provide enough support for the game's constant lateral movement. Beginners should buy a lightweight, oversize racket, which will improve their chances of making contact with the ball, says Coyne. If your racket's too heavy, your arm will get tired. But if it's too light, you'll be waving it like a wand, not learning proper strokes.

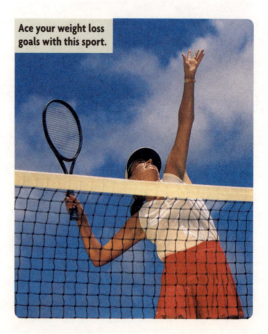

Ace your weight loss goals with this sport.

Walking

What could be simpler than putting one foot in front of the other? That's all there is to walking. You don't need fancy equipment, a health club membership, or even good weather. Indoors, you can walk on a treadmill or stride around a mall. Outside, the sky's the limit. And though it's easy, it's no wimpy workout.

Walking can give you all the rewards of aerobic exercise without putting much stress on your knees, hips, and back. A walking routine can help lower your risk of heart disease, reduce your cholesterol and blood pressure, speed up fat loss, and increase muscle tone, says Rosemary Agostini, MD, clinical associate professor of orthopedics at the University of Washington and staff physician at the Virginia Mason Sports Medicine Center, both in Seattle.

WALKING STATS

CALORIES BURNED*	BODY-SHAPING BONUS
100 per mile	Tones abs, hips, thighs, and buttocks

* Based on a 150-lb woman. If you weigh more, you'll burn more calories; if you weigh less, you'll burn fewer.

WORKOUTS

Beginner Walk for 20 minutes, 6 or 7 days a week for 2 weeks.

Intermediate Walk for 25 minutes, 6 or 7 days a week; increase walking time by 10% increments each week until you reach 40 minutes.

Experienced Continue to increase walking time by 10% until you reach 45 to 60 minutes, 6 or 7 days a week. If you don't need to lose body fat, you can walk 20 to 30 minutes, 3 days a week to stay fit.

Beginners should aim for a level of exertion equivalent to a 6 or 7 on a scale of 1 to 10, advises Bonnie Stein, a nationally known race-walking instructor and coach in Redington Shores, FL. You should be able to carry on a conversation without being short of breath. As you develop endurance and lose weight, increase your walking time and the intensity by aiming for an exertion level of 7 or 8.

part 3

stretch it out!

66 **Tone Up and Get Flexible Fast**
Stretch out your fitness benefits
with this daily routine

74 **Essential Stretches for
Stress Relief**
These fluid moves will help you
stand up straight with a smile

79 **7 Moves to a More
Balanced You**
Ease achy muscles and an anxious mind
with this ancient discipline

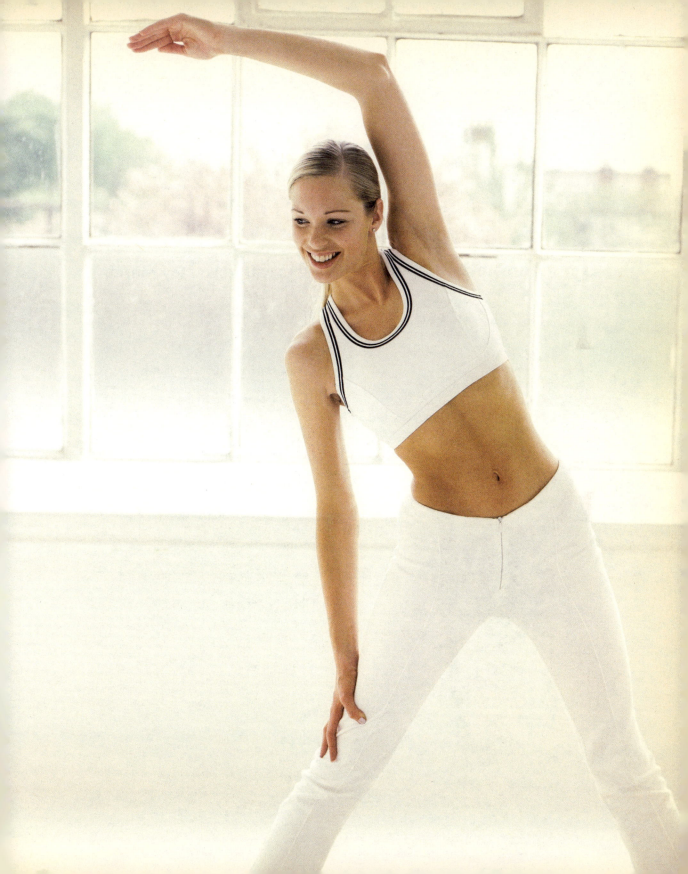

CHAPTER 9

Tone Up and Get Flexible Fast

Stretch out your fitness benefits with this daily routine

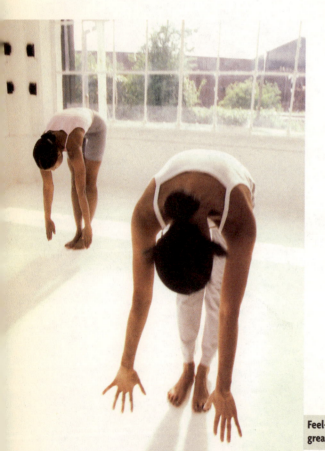

Be honest. Even when you're faithful to your cardio and strength training, you often cheat on your stretching, sometimes to the point of skipping it entirely. You're hardly alone. The American Council on Exercise named "neglecting to stretch" the mistake folks make most often while getting in shape. And that's a shame, because stretching takes no more than 10 minutes a day, and the pay-offs are enormous.

Feel-good moves for a great-looking body.

The Big Benefits of a Limber Body

We all know we're supposed to stretch. But few of us appreciate all the benefits lengthening our muscles and connective tissue has to offer. Here are some of the rewards flexibility can provide.

Longer, "looser" muscles. Stretching will make you feel better, especially if you're working out and weight training. Muscles remember the last thing you do. And if the last thing you've done is contract them over and over while running, bicycling, or pressing dumbbells, they'll end up tighter and shorter. Stretch them every day, and you'll feel limber and comfortable.

Tension relief. Every muscle in your body contains "stretch receptors" that keep a constant dialogue going with your brain about your overall level of tension. When your muscles are chronically tight, your body is thrown out of alignment, creating muscular imbalances and poor posture. That notifies your brain that your body is under constant stress. Can you say tension headache?

Better performance. Stretching makes your body perform better. You'll gain a greater range of motion, so you can generate more force. Your stride will be longer, your golf swing will be stronger, and you'll think nothing of taking the stairs two at a time. Flexible muscles also help prevent muscle soreness.

Look like a dancer. Yoga, Pilates, and other flexibility-producing exercises are popular with dancers (and people who want to look like dancers) because well-stretched muscles appear leaner and longer than shortened, constantly contracted muscles. Stretching also undoes a lot of the postural damage we do even when we're not working out.

It's all good. Stretching has some hidden psychological benefits. Just as chronically tight muscles send a signal to your brain that you're under constant stress, chronically relaxed muscles send the opposite message, telling your brain that everything is okay. That can make you feel less stressed out even when things are crazy. Plus, when done properly, stretching simply feels good.

Simple Daily Stretches

Stretching is most effective when it's done after working out, when your muscles are warm and pliable. Some women prefer stretching during a special time of day, such as in the evening while watching television. That's okay too. Just be sure to warm up with a little activity such as walking or jogging in place first. Stretching when your muscles are cold leaves you vulnerable to injury.

These stretches, recommended by Carol Espel, MS, exercise physiologist and general manager at Equinox Fitness Club in Scarsdale, NY, hit every major muscle group in the body. For each one, hold the stretch for 10 to 30 seconds, breathing deeply all the time.

When your muscles are chronically tight, your body is thrown out of alignment, creating muscular imbalances and poor posture. Can you say tension headache?

HAMSTRINGS

Lie on your back with your legs bent and both feet on the floor. Straighten and raise your left leg. Gently pull your thigh toward your body, and hold. If you can't reach your leg, loop a towel over your foot and, with a slight bend at the knee, gently pull your leg toward your chest. Repeat with your right leg.

[1]

[2]

[3]

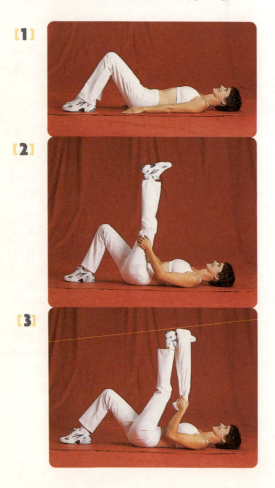

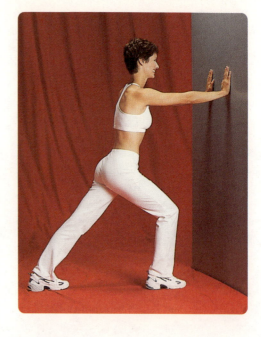

CALVES

Stand facing a wall, with your right foot about 18 inches from the wall and your left foot about 2 feet behind it. Place your hands against the wall for support, and lean forward while pressing your left heel to the floor. Switch legs.

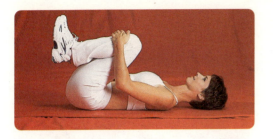

LOWER BACK

Lie on your back, and pull both knees to your chest. Keep your upper body relaxed on the floor.

QUADRICEPS AND HIP FLEXORS

Put your left hand on a wall. Bending your right knee, bring your right foot toward your buttocks; hold it in place with your right hand. Keep your knees together, and do not arch your back. Repeat with your left leg, putting your right hand on the wall.

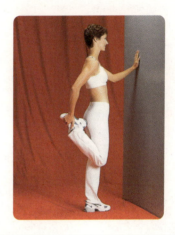

TRICEPS AND SIDES

Stand straight, and raise your left arm over your head; bend the elbow, and drop your hand toward the middle of your back. With your right hand, gently pull your left elbow to the right. Tilt your body to the right to stretch the muscles in your side. Keep your stomach tight. Repeat with your right arm.

[1]   [2]

CHEST

Stand with your feet shoulder-width apart and knees slightly bent. Clasp your hands behind your back with your palms facing in toward your body. Slowly push your chest forward, keeping your back and abdomen stable. (If this movement is uncomfortable, do the stretch without your hands touching.) You can lean forward slightly, but don't allow yourself to become pitched forward.

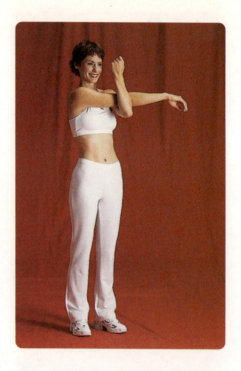

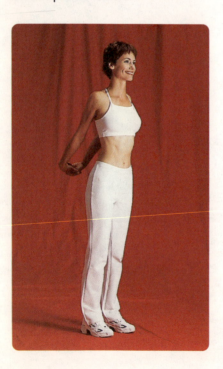

UPPER BACK AND SHOULDERS

Cross your right arm in front of your chest. With the opposite arm, gently pull your right arm toward your body, and hold. Repeat with your left arm.

UPPER BACK

Clasp your hands in front of you with your palms facing away. Round your back, drop your chin to your chest, relax your shoulders, and press your hands forward.

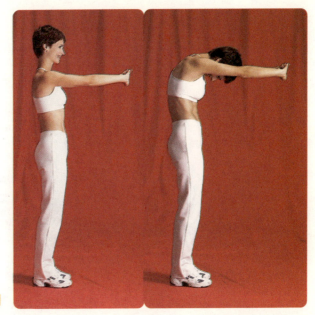

[1]   [2]

HIPS

Lie on your back with your legs straight. Bend your right leg so it crosses over the left, keeping your foot near your left knee. Using your left hand, gently press your right knee toward the floor until you feel a stretch in your right hip and buttocks. Hold, then repeat with your left leg.

[1]

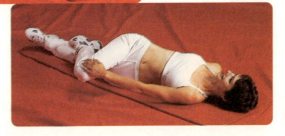

[2]

How to Get a Good Stretch

Stretching is as simple to do as bending and breathing. Before you begin, here are six rules of thumb to keep in mind as you reach for a longer, more limber body.

Stretch warm.

As eager as you may be to begin, don't just leap out of bed and start doing splits. Your muscles need to have some blood pumping through them and be warm and at least somewhat supple to be stretched safely and effectively. Always warm up for a few minutes by jogging in place, or just 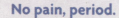 swing your arms and legs a little bit, before asking your muscles to lengthen.

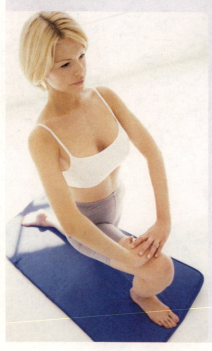

No pain, period.

It's tempting to try to speed your progress by stretching just a little farther than is comfortably possible, but resist the urge to do so. Muscles are equipped with a safety mechanism called a stretch reflex. When you push a muscle too far, this sensor kicks in, and the muscle responds with a reflexive contraction, shortening the muscle to protect it from overextending the joint. This is not the response you want when you're trying to lengthen tight muscles. Stretch only to the point where you feel gentle tension, then stop, and hold the stretch. As you continue to stretch regularly, you'll be able to reach progressively farther and farther before you feel that tension. Becoming flexible means being able to stretch your muscles without pain.

Maybe before, definitely after.

Most fitness professionals will tell you to stretch before and after any physical activity, which is great advice. But like most folks, you'll probably never do it. Stretching before exercise means taking 5 minutes to warm up, stopping, stretching, then resuming activity—something most people don't find practical. Plus, a recent study of more than 2,600 Army recruits found that, contrary to conventional wisdom, stretching before exercise didn't alter injury rate during activity. But stretching *after* exercising was still important to keep muscles performing at their optimal range of motion.

The take-home advice is to warm up at a light pace, gradually increasing your intensity and purposefully stretching out your movements to boost your circulation and get your muscles ready for activity. Exercise as normal, cool down when you're done, then spend 5 to 10 minutes gently stretching the muscles you've just used before hitting the showers. It's a natural progression that'll leave you feeling great all over.

Slow and steady.

Don't bounce while you stretch! No matter how much this point is repeated, some people are still locked into that "bobbing and stretching" mode. It's counterproductive and can cause injury. Keep your stretches slow and steady, holding each one for 10 to 30 seconds.

Breathe.

It sounds simple, but it's easy to forget. Breathe deeply during your stretches. If you find yourself holding your breath, you're pushing too hard.

Sneak it in.

Ideally, you should stretch every day. If that's not realistic, at least stretch the muscles you use on the days you work them. You can make this a no-brainer by simply working your stretches into your routine. On weight training days, for instance, stretch the muscles you're working in between sets. So after a set of chest presses, stretch your pectorals; after squats, stretch your legs. It's a more efficient use of your time, and you'll lift better because your muscles are more limber.

CHAPTER 10

Essential Stretches for Stress Relief

These fluid moves will help you stand up straight with a smile

Next time you're fretting about a family feud or frazzled over ever-looming deadlines, take a peek in the nearest reflective surface. Sloping shoulders. Hunched back. Furrowed forehead. Hardly a pretty picture. That's what too much stress can do. Your muscles tighten, which restricts bloodflow. Over time, this can create a buildup of calcifications (those hard knots most of us have in our upper back), giving us a hunched-over, aged look, as well as restricting our movement. The poor posture most of us walk around sporting, especially when we're stressed out, only makes matters worse.

Round-the-clock relaxation—guaranteed!

24-Hour Stress Relief

Following are a day's worth of anxiety-busting stretches recommended by Jo Fasen, PT, orthopedic clinical specialist at the Rehabilitation Institute of Chicago's Center for Spine, Sports, and Occupational Rehabilitation. Do them all for a stress-relieving, invigorating routine, or do individual stretches for specific problems such as sore shoulders or an achy back. If you don't see improvement after a month of consistent stretching, or you still have pain, see a physical therapist.

THE "DE-SLUMP" STRETCH

(WHERE YOU'LL FEEL IT: **chest, shoulders, upper back**)

Sit on the edge of a chair with your pelvis tilted slightly forward and your legs spread as wide as comfortable. Slide your chin back so that your ears align over your shoulders. Lift your chest, and squeeze your shoulder blades together and down away from your ears. Reach both arms wide and slightly behind you. Your palms should be facing forward, fingers spread. Don't arch your lower back. Hold, then repeat.

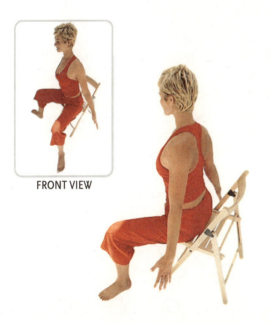

FRONT VIEW

THE "WALK WITH CONFIDENCE" STRETCH

(WHERE YOU'LL FEEL IT: **front of hips**)

Stand with your feet a few inches apart, then move one leg about 1 to 2 feet forward. Bend your knees, making sure your front knee is directly over the ankle. Your back heel will come off the floor. Keep your posture upright as you tuck in your abdomen and butt and tilt your pelvis. Hold, then repeat. This stretch also relieves hip pain.

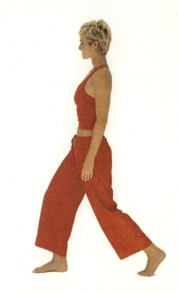

THE HUNCHBACK REMOVER

(WHERE YOU'LL FEEL IT: **sides of your neck**)

While sitting in a chair, hook your left hand, palm facing you, on the back of the seat next to your left buttock. Hold on as you lean forward. Keep your shoulders back, and drop your right ear toward your right shoulder. Then roll your chin forward, and hold. Switch hands, and repeat on the other side. This stretch also eases neck pain.

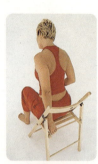

REAR VIEW

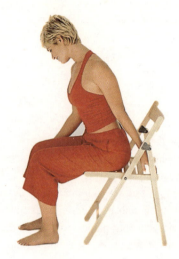

Customize Your Routine

If you're not doing the entire routine, Jo Fasen, PT, recommends that you choose stretches that correspond to the stresses you chronically place on your body.

DESK JOB OR AVID CYCLIST: To reverse the position you're in most of the time, do extension exercises that open the chest and the front of the hips and that lengthen the back of the thighs and spine. Try the De-Slump and Goodbye Achy Back stretches.

ON YOUR FEET ALL DAY OR A WALKER OR RUNNER: You'll want to relieve those muscles that have been used all day, namely the calves, front of thighs, and back. Try the Stand Up Straight and Goodbye Achy Back stretches.

NEW MOTHER: You may have a rounded posture due to the demands of breastfeeding and carrying your baby. If this is you, try the De-Slump and Hunchback Remover stretches.

OLDER ADULTS: You'll need to stretch your chest (to prevent hunching over) and your hips and calves (to optimize walking and balance). Try the De-Slump and Walk with Confidence stretches.

THE "STAND UP STRAIGHT" STRETCH

(WHERE YOU'LL FEEL IT: **abs, sides, and back**)

Stand straight with your feet shoulder-width apart, hips facing forward, and abs tight. Gently twist your trunk to the right, and hold. Return to the starting position, and repeat to the left side. Next, gently lean to the right as you reach your left arm up toward the ceiling; curve it slightly overhead, palm down. Keep your shoulders down and relaxed. Hold, then repeat to the left side.

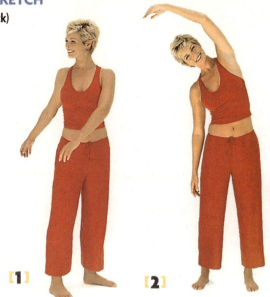

[1]   **[2]**

10 Commandments of De-Stress Stretching

1. Follow a program that is specific to your activities and needs.

2. Stretch regularly, at least three times a week.

3. Warm up before stretching.

4. Stretch only to the point where you feel tension in the belly of the muscle, not pain in the joint.

5. Hold each stretch for 15 to 60 seconds.

6. Do each stretch two to four times.

7. Stay relaxed.

8. Breathe throughout the stretch.

9. Progress in a slow, controlled manner.

10. Don't bounce.

THE "GOODBYE ACHY BACK" STRETCH

(WHERE YOU'LL FEEL IT: **butt, thighs, chest, upper back, shoulders, and abs**)

Stand with your feet shoulder-width apart and your abs tight. Keeping your back straight, bend at the hips and knees, reaching your hands through your legs, if comfortable. Hold. Caution: Don't do this if you have back pain.

Next, use your hips to straighten up, reaching your arms overhead and slightly behind you. Hold. Don't arch your back. Repeat the entire sequence. This stretch also improves posture and muscle tone.

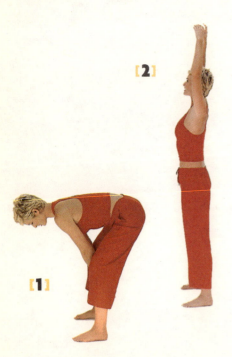

Aging Gracefully

Daily stretching is like stashing spare change in a savings account. You won't see big dividends on a daily basis, but in 30 years you'll really reap the benefits.

Starting in your 30s, your body's connective tissues (muscles, tendons, and ligaments) start to shorten and tighten, losing elasticity, says Marilyn Moffat, PhD, PT, past president of the American Physical Therapy Association and professor of physical therapy at New York University in New York City. Making matters worse, chronic poor posture (such as slumping while you sit, something we're *all* guilty of) causes tight muscles and constricted bloodflow, which can leave you with a limited range of motion and the hunched-over appearance of a little old lady.

But despite the damage you've done, and no matter how old you are, flexibility can be regained by stretching regularly—and improvement can be seen within weeks. When you stretch, you actually lengthen the muscles and tendons.

This is what increasing flexibility means. When a muscle is flexible, it enables the joint to completely flex, extend, and move in multiple directions (known as range of motion), whether it's to throw a Frisbee or turn a car's steering wheel.

The end result is that regular stretchers look, act, and feel younger than their years. In one study, people 60 and older increased their walking speed by simply stretching regularly—nothing else. Now those are results worth banking on!

CHAPTER 11

7 Moves to a More Balanced You

Ease achy muscles and an anxious mind with this ancient discipline

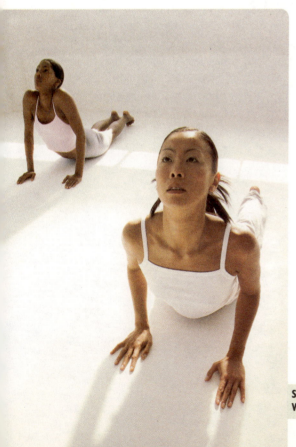

**Stress?
What stress?**

Yoga has taken the US by storm, and with good reason. This 3,000-year-old exercise is just what most tensed-up Americans need for their muscles below their neck—as well as that one between their ears!

For a refresher: Yoga is a series of postures, called asanas, that you hold while breathing deeply. Yoga, which means to unite or yoke, was originally designed to connect the body and the spirit. It relaxes tight muscles and ligaments, reduces stress, and improves balance, flexibility, strength, and coordination. People who practice yoga regularly also praise its mind-calming benefits. Done regularly, yoga can leave you feeling centered and peaceful in a pretty stressful world.

Find Your Flow

Before beginning yoga practice, remember that it's all about expanding your body's natural flow. It's not about forcing yourself into painful positions so you can look as good or better than the pictures in this book or the yoga goddesses you see folded up like pretzels in the gym. Everyone's body is different, so there's no shame in adapting postures to suit your needs. Move into a pose only as far as is comfortable. Stretching farther than is comfortable can stress your connective tissues and actually make them weaker rather than stronger over time. Stop when you feel mild discomfort. And relax; flexibility will come.

The following yoga and yoga-inspired poses are a good introduction to this ancient discipline. Hold each pose for 15 to 60 seconds (depending on your experience and comfort level), breathing deeply throughout.

WARRIOR

Stand tall with your feet about hip-width apart. Take a giant step forward with your right foot, bending that knee. (Be sure your knee does not jut out over your toes.) Turn your left foot to the side so your left arch faces the heel of your right foot. Raise your arms over your head, your palms facing each other, lifting your chin slightly. Hold, then switch sides.

DOWNWARD DOG

Position yourself on the floor on your hands and knees, your feet flexed. Press your hands and feet into the floor, raising your hips toward the ceiling. Your body should look like an upside-down V. Keep lifting your tailbone toward the ceiling as you lower your heels to the floor as far as comfortably possible.

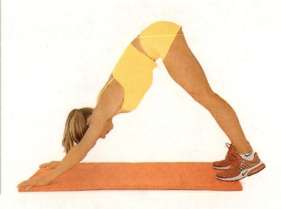

CAT

Kneel on your hands and knees with your head, neck, and back in alignment. Keeping your shoulders relaxed, lower your chin toward your chest, pull in your belly, and round your back, like a cat arching. Hold, then slowly return to the starting position.

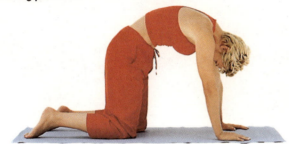

Yoga Do's and Don'ts

Perform these three popular moves <u>without</u> these common mistakes

Yoga is best learned through a class, where you can receive individual instruction, but that's not always possible. Here's how to correct common mistakes, avoid injury, and get the most for your yoga moves.

WARRIOR

Do: Keep your knee over your ankle.　　**Don't:** Let your knee jut forward.

DOWNWARD DOG

Do: Roll your shoulders out.　　**Don't:** Jam and roll your shoulders in.

COBRA

Do: Lift through the top of your head to extend your spine.　　**Don't:** Collapse into your shoulders.

COW

Kneel on your hands and knees with your head, neck, and back in alignment. Arch your back, creating an inward curve with your butt lifted toward the ceiling and your head looking up just slightly. Hold, then return to the starting position.

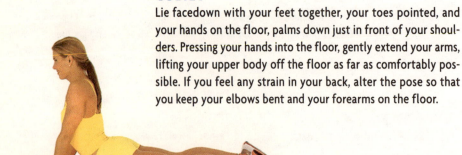

Done regularly, yoga can leave you feeling centered and peaceful in a pretty stressful world.

COBRA

Lie facedown with your feet together, your toes pointed, and your hands on the floor, palms down just in front of your shoulders. Pressing your hands into the floor, gently extend your arms, lifting your upper body off the floor as far as comfortably possible. If you feel any strain in your back, alter the pose so that you keep your elbows bent and your forearms on the floor.

LYING ROTATION

Lie on the floor on your right side with your right arm bent underneath your head. Bend both legs so you're comfortable. Imagine that you're lying on a big clock. Extend your left arm in front of you on the floor as if it's a clock hand pointing to 9 o'clock. Slowly rotate your arm toward 12 o'clock. As you hit 1 o'clock, you'll start to roll back, but keep your hips and legs where they are. Keeping your arm on the floor, rotate it through all the numbers on the clock (your palm will flip up momentarily behind you), over your hips, and back to the starting position.

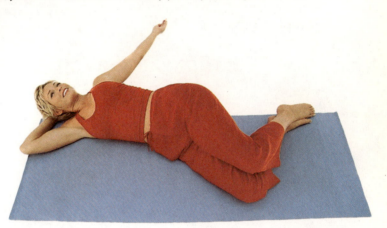

CHILD'S POSE

Kneel with your toes pointed behind you. Sit back onto your heels, and lower your chest to your thighs. Stretch your arms overhead, and rest your palms and forehead on the floor (or as close as comfortable).

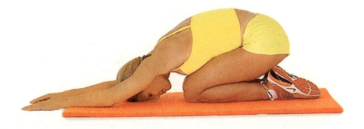

part 4

eat to lose!

86 **Sorting Out the Carb Confusion**
Low-carbohydrate eating made
safe, fast, and easy!

96 **Pick Your Protein Wisely**
Smart cuts can make meat a healthy and
tasty part of your weight loss plan

100 **Welcome Back Fat!**
The savory flavors you love can *finally* be part of
a healthy weight loss diet!

104 **Customize Your Weight Loss Plan**
Get the body you've always wanted eating
foods you love

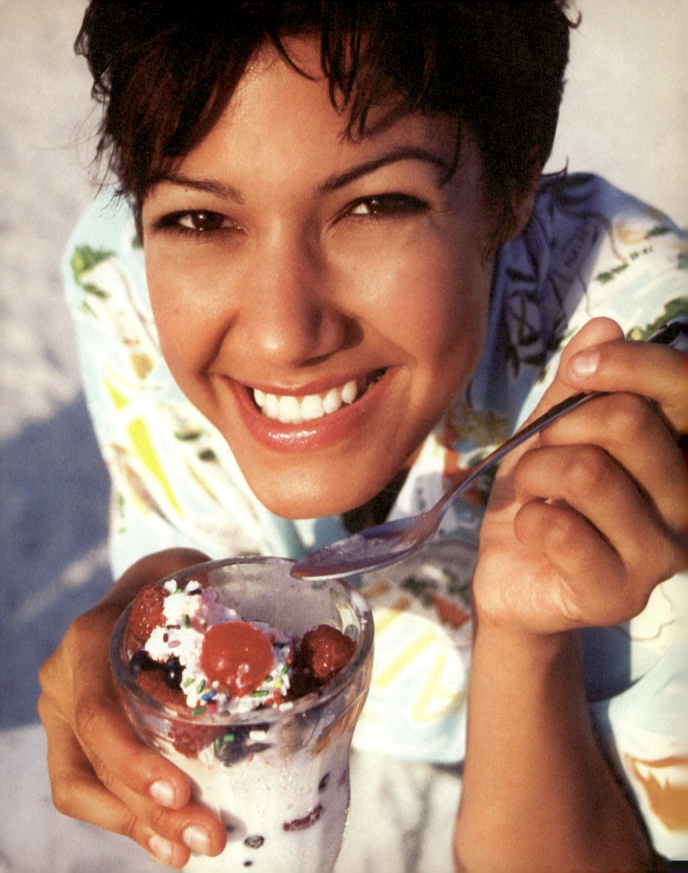

CHAPTER 12

Sorting Out the Carb Confusion

Low-carbohydrate eating made safe, fast, and easy!

By now, we *all* know someone who's dropped three sizes eating cheeseburgers (without the bun), bacon, and steak 'n eggs. You're probably smart enough to know these extreme high-protein diets can't be healthy. But let's face it: You're more than a little envious of the weight loss. Maybe you're even tempted to stock up on some sausage yourself. Well, while you should definitely hold the hot dogs, we at *Prevention* believe that cutting carbs and pumping up protein, when planned wisely, may be the most effective and satisfying way to lose weight and keep it off!

Have your bread, and lose pounds too.

We certainly aren't saying you should eliminate carbohydrates altogether. And we're not saying you can eat all the bacon and cream you want. What we're saying is that the majority of your calories—your daily diet—should come from lean protein foods such as chicken, healthy fats such as olive oil, and yes, good-for-you carbohydrates such as vegetables and whole grains.

In addition to weight loss, family doctors have been surprised to see that the people who have followed this remarkable approach have reduced their risk of heart disease, diabetes, and cancer while also boosting their energy levels and getting a new outlook on life.

How Good Carbs Got a Bad Rap

Let's be clear. Carbohydrates are *not* evil. Fact is, you can't live without them. Carbohydrates are one of three basic macronutrients needed to sustain life (the other two are protein and fat). But eating too many carbohydrates, especially refined carbohydrates, can cause you to gain weight and can adversely affect your health.

Carbohydrates encompass a broad range of sugars, starches, and fibers. There are two general classes of carbs: refined and unrefined. Refined carbohydrates are essentially refined sugars and refined flours. Generally speaking, refined carbohydrates are less healthy. Numerous studies demonstrate the relationship of these less-healthy carbohydrates to type 2 diabetes, heart disease, and even some kinds of cancer.

Unrefined carbohydrates are the kind found in whole grains, beans, fruits, and many vegetables. Unrefined carbs are usually more healthy because they include two kinds of fiber: soluble and insoluble. Fiber is extremely important for

The Great Carb Blocker Debate
Tantalizing promise, controversial results

As more people turn to low-carb living, supplements called carb blockers (such as Carb Trapper, Carb Cutter, and Carb-X) are popping up on store shelves everywhere. The claim: One or two tablets with a meal can block the absorption of about 400 calories' worth of bread, pasta, or potatoes.

But do they really work? The main ingredients are bean and wheat germ extracts thought to stop carbohydrate absorption by inhibiting a digestive enzyme that breaks down starch. If starch passes through you undigested, you should lose weight.

That's the theory, but the truth is this: There's only a little evidence that they might work. In the '80s, several studies showed that the bean extract had no effect on calorie absorption or body weight.

But recently, however, researchers at the Mayo Clinic found that higher doses of bean extract (4,000 to 6,000 mg) and wheat germ extract (4,000 mg) slowed carbohydrate digestion. But these higher doses are not available in commercial carb blockers, plus no one knows whether they cause weight loss over time.

Your Whole Grain Guide

Check this smart-carb list before you stock your shelves

Shopping for whole grains? Make it a point to bring home these brands.

BREAD

Alvarado St. Sprouted
   Sourdough Bread
Goya Corn Tortillas
Matthew's Whole Wheat
   English Muffins
Mestemacher Three Grain Bread
Mestemacher Whole Rye Bread
   with Muesli
Pepperidge Farm 100% Stone Ground
   Whole Wheat Bread
Thomas' Sahara 100% Whole Wheat
   Pita Bread
Wonder Stone Ground 100%
   Whole Wheat Bread

CEREAL

Arrowhead Mills Steel Cut Oats
General Mills Cheerios
General Mills Wheat Chex
Kellogg's Frosted Mini-Wheats
Post Bran Flakes
Post Raisin Bran
Quaker Instant Oatmeal
Quaker Old Fashioned Oats
Quaker Quick 1 Minute Oats

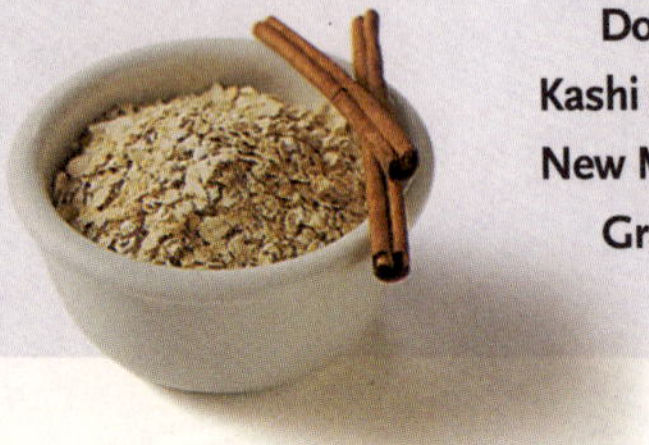

CRACKERS

Ak-mak Stone Ground Sesame Cracker
Kavli Hearty Thick Crispbread
Ryvita Sesame Rye Crispbread
Wasa Hearty Rye Original Crispbread
Whole Foods Baked Woven Wheats

PASTA

Annie's Whole Wheat Shells & Cheddar
DeCecco Whole Wheat Linguine
Fantastic Whole Wheat Couscous
Hodgson Mill Whole Wheat Bow Tie
Hodgson Mill Whole Wheat Lasagna

RICE

Fantastic Brown Basmati Rice
Kraft Minute Instant Brown Rice
Lundberg Family Farms Wehani
   Brown Rice
Success 10 Minute Brown Rice
Uncle Ben's Instant Brown Rice
Wegmans Quick Cook Spanish
   Brown Rice

SNACKS

Bearitos Tortilla Chips
Health Valley Healthy Chips
   Double Chocolate Cookies
Kashi Seven Whole Grains & Sesame
New Morning Organic Cinnamon
   Grahams

weight management because it makes you feel full so you don't overeat, and it helps slow down your body's absorption of carbohydrate foods. Fiber also helps stabilize blood sugar levels and may help reduce the risk of heart disease.

All carbohydrates are eventually converted by your body into glucose (blood sugar). One hundred percent of the carbohydrate you eat turns into glucose, but only 58% of the protein and about 10% of the fat you eat is converted to glucose.

The Carbohydrate/ Weight Connection

So how does a carb-heavy diet make you heavy? If you eat excessive amounts of quickly absorbed refined carbohydrates, you upset your body's precise balance of blood sugar. Simply put, eating too many carbohydrate grams may cause a situation where more glucose becomes available to the cells than the body needs. You gain weight because the excess glucose gets turned into fat.

Once the glucose is safely stored away as fat, your blood sugar drops, and—you guessed it— you start to feel hungry again. If, like many Americans, you eat a lot of refined carbohydrates such as soft drinks and candy bars (or even pretzels and crackers), you are feeding a vicious circle in your body that never really satisfies your hunger because you get only short-term relief.

Plus, most refined carbohydrate foods are low in fiber. As mentioned earlier, eating fiber-rich foods gives you a sense of fullness. On the other hand, eating low-fiber, simple carbohydrate foods leaves you feeling constantly hungry. This cycle may help to explain why sugar seems to have an addictive quality and how carbohydrate-rich meals may lead to excess weight.

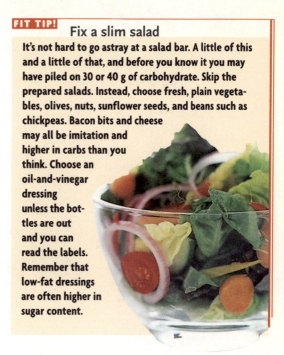

FIT TIP! Fix a slim salad

It's not hard to go astray at a salad bar. A little of this and a little of that, and before you know it you may have piled on 30 or 40 g of carbohydrate. Skip the prepared salads. Instead, choose fresh, plain vegetables, olives, nuts, sunflower seeds, and beans such as chickpeas. Bacon bits and cheese may all be imitation and higher in carbs than you think. Choose an oil-and-vinegar dressing unless the bottles are out and you can read the labels. Remember that low-fat dressings are often higher in sugar content.

By eating less of the quickly absorbed carbohydrates, keeping moderate amounts of lean proteins and healthy fats in your diet, and getting a reasonable amount of physical activity, you set the stage for safe and effective weight loss.

What's more, with an emphasis on unrefined carbohydrate foods you will get more fiber, vitamins, and minerals to help slow the absorption of carbs into your bloodstream. Slow, gradual absorption will prevent your body from producing excess glucose. The extra protein and healthy fats in this diet will also help satisfy your appetite, so you'll experience less hunger and be less likely to get sudden urges for sweets or extra portions. All of this adds up to an easier and healthier way to shed pounds!

At-a-Glance Guide to Cutting Carbs

Use these visual cues to control portions and shave pounds fast

In reasonable portion sizes, no carbs are off-limits. The trick is knowing what a sensible serving is in a world where food servings have grown to astronomical proportions. Here's a guide to help you avoid sneaky oversized carbs. Choose the foods that most closely match the serving sizes on the left, and save up to hundreds of calories a day.

CHOOSE THIS SIZE	INSTEAD OF THIS SIZE
MUFFIN 2 oz $2^3/_4$" diameter 2" high Size of a small apple 169 cal, 7 g fat 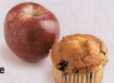	**MEGA-MUFFIN** 10–12 oz $4^1/_2$" diameter $3^1/_2$" high Size of a medium grapefruit 850–1,020 cal, 34–41 g fat
COOKIE $^1/_3$ oz Size of half a yo-yo 48 cal, 2 g fat 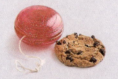	**SUPERSIZE COOKIE** 4 oz Size of a teacup saucer 544 cal, 26 g fat 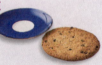
CINNAMON ROLL WITH FROSTING 1 oz Size of a tangerine 108 cal, 4 g fat 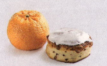	**GIANT CINNAMON ROLL** 7.5 oz Size of a cereal bowl 670 cal, 34 g fat
BAGEL 2 oz 3" diameter No wider than a credit card and about $^1/_2$" high 157 cal, 1 g fat 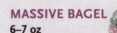	**MASSIVE BAGEL** 6–7 oz 5" diameter Size of a stack of 30 CDs (out of their cases, of course) 468–546 cal, 5–6 g fat

CHOOSE THIS SIZE	INSTEAD OF THIS SIZE
PRETZELS 3" wide 2½" long Size of a makeup compact 160 cal, 1 g fat (per 1.5-oz serving, or 4 pretzels)	**LARGE SOFT PRETZEL** 7" wide 6" long Size of a dessert plate 270–510 cal, 1–13 g fat (depending on the flavor)
HAMBURGER BUN 1.5 oz 3" diameter 1¼" high Size of a 6-oz tuna can 123 cal, 2 g fat	**BIG BUN** 2.8 oz 4½" diameter 2" high Size of a stack of 30 CDs (out of their cases, of course) 210 cal, 5 g fat
PASTA SERVING 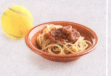 ½ cup* Size of a tennis ball 94 cal, 1 g fat (with tomato sauce) * ½ cup is considered a starch food exchange in many diets; however, 1 or 1½ cups is a realistic serving size	**HUGE RESTAURANT PASTA SERVING** 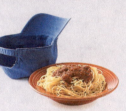 3½ cups Enough to fill the inside of a baseball cap 849 cal, 17 g fat (with tomato sauce)
BROWNIE 1.5 oz 2" square ¾" thick Size of a Nabisco Oreo cookie, except square and slightly thicker 177 cal, 9 g fat	**LARGE BAKERY BROWNIE** 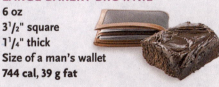 6 oz 3½" square 1¼" thick Size of a man's wallet 744 cal, 39 g fat

Real Food, Real Success

The other reason our smart low-carb diet is so successful is that it takes a whole new approach by starting with your current eating patterns. Unlike a strict diet that forces you to empty your fridge and cupboards into the trash, smart low-carb eating includes many of your favorite foods such as pasta, grains, and even potatoes. No food is completely off-limits. You can start immediately or gradually adopt the smart low-carb plan over time.

Even better, smart low-carb is a plan you can—and should—stick with for life. Years of research and good science show that this method won't just bring you weight loss success; it will also help you prevent a bevy of diseases.

Researchers at the University of Illinois compared the widely recommended USDA diet (a high-carb plan) with a lower-carbohydrate diet that is very similar to the one recommended here. Interestingly, both diets had the same number of calories. In the study, 24 women who were overweight ate 1,700 calories a day for 10 weeks. One group ate according to the USDA Food Guide Pyramid (55% carbohydrates, 15% protein, and 30% fat). The other group ate a lower-carb, higher-protein diet (40% carbohydrates, 30% protein, and

DO JUST ONE THING!

Sack the sugar, and keep off pounds for good

In a society that's saturated in soft drinks and powdered doughnuts, sugar can be a major diet disaster. Just ask Betty Carlucci, 60. Betty had maintained a healthy weight most of her adult life—until she hit menopause, when she found herself bowled over by sweet cravings. "It seemed that if I ate anything with even a little sugar in it, I got more and more hungry. And this really put on the pounds—40 of them!" she recalls.

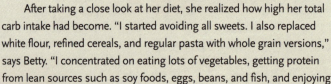

After taking a close look at her diet, she realized how high her total carb intake had become. "I started avoiding all sweets. I also replaced white flour, refined cereals, and regular pasta with whole grain versions," says Betty. "I concentrated on eating lots of vegetables, getting protein from lean sources such as soy foods, eggs, beans, and fish, and enjoying fresh fruit now and then."

The result: She not only dropped the weight she'd gained, but she picked up added energy and stamina, both of which she needs to keep up with her young grandchildren. "I enjoy my food more now. And I'm truly enjoying the commitment and discipline of taking care of myself," says Betty.

Science shows that a low-carb approach, when planned wisely, may be one of the most effective and satisfying ways to lose weight and keep it off.

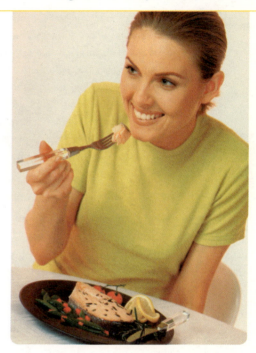

30% fat). After 10 weeks, the women in both groups lost about 16 lb. But the women on the lower-carbohydrate diet had a more healthy weight loss. They lost about 12 lb of body fat and just over 1 lb of muscle mass. Those who followed the USDA diet lost only 10 lb of body fat and a surprising 3 lb of metabolism-revving muscle mass. This means that the low-carb, high-protein diet was almost twice as effective for long-term weight loss because the women who followed it burned calories more efficiently.

At the end of the study, the women on the low-carb diet also had increased levels of beneficial thyroid hormones, suggesting that their metabolisms went up—another plus for burning calories. One more bonus with the low-carb diet: The women following this plan experienced a sharp reduction in triglycerides (fat in the blood) and a slight increase in high-density lipoprotein (HDL, the beneficial type of cholesterol), which improved their overall heart health.

Another study suggests that you may even be able to eat more calories on the smart low-carb diet and *still* lose weight. Researchers at the Albert Einstein College of Medicine in the Bronx looked at caloric intake of overweight teenagers following a low-carbohydrate plan compared with that of teens on a low-fat plan over a period of 12 weeks. Although the teenagers on the low-carb plan ate an average of 600 calories more per day than the other teens, they lost an average of 11 lb more. The teens on the low-fat plan ate fewer calories but lost an average of only 10 lb, while those on the low-carb plan ate more calories and lost around 20 lb. This study suggests that calories may not be the only deciding factor in weight loss; what *kind* of calories may be even more important. That's where this plan comes in. (See chapter 15 for the full Smart Low-Carb plan.)

Fast Carb, Slow Carb

Eating according to the Glycemic Index can help you lose weight

Choosing foods with a low glycemic index (GI) can help you shed pounds faster. That's because low-GI foods are slowly digested and help prevent the spikes in blood sugar that can cause food cravings and lead to weight gain. Low-GI foods have a ranking of 55 or lower. High-GI foods have a ranking of 56 or higher. If you choose a high-GI food, try to combine it with a low-GI food or a food that is high in protein or fat. This will slow the absorption of the high-GI food and prevent your blood sugar from rising rapidly. Foods printed in green are high-GI foods that you need not avoid; these foods, such as carrots and watermelon, contain important nutrients besides carbohydrates. Foods printed in red are low-GI foods that are best eaten sparingly; these foods, such as potato chips, are high in fat or calories and don't offer much else nutritionally.

FOOD	GI
BAKED GOODS	
French bread	95
Waffle	76
Graham cracker	74
Kaiser roll	73
Bagel	72
Corn tortilla	70
Melba toast	70
White bread	70
Whole wheat bread	69
Taco shell	68
Angel food cake	67
Croissant	67
Stoned wheat thins	67
100% whole rye bread	65
Rye crispbread	65
Bran muffin	60
Whole wheat pita	57
Oatmeal cookie	55
Pumpernickel bread	41
CEREALS	
Puffed rice	88
Cornflakes	84
Puffed wheat	74
Cream of Wheat	70
Shredded wheat	69
Quick-cooking oats	66
Old-fashioned oats	59
Oat bran	55
All-Bran	42
GRAINS	
Instant rice	91
Millet	71
Cornmeal	68
White rice	68
Couscous	65
Brown rice	55
Buckwheat	54
Bulgur	48
Parboiled rice	47
Pearled barley	26
PASTAS	
Brown rice pasta	92
Gnocchi	68
Boxed macaroni and cheese	64
Rice vermicelli	58
Durum spaghetti	55
Cheese tortellini	50
Linguine	46
White spaghetti	41
Meat-filled ravioli	39
Whole grain spaghetti	37

Vermicelli	35
Fettuccine	32
Bean threads	26

LEGUMES

Fava beans	79
Canned kidney beans	52
Canned baked beans	48
Canned pinto beans	45
Black-eyed peas	42
Canned chickpeas	42
Chickpeas	33
Lima beans	32
Yellow split peas	32
Butter beans	31
Green lentils	30
Kidney beans	27
Red lentils	26
Soybeans	18

DAIRY AND ICE CREAMS

Tofu frozen dessert	115
Ice cream	61
Sweetened, fruited yogurt	33
Fat-free milk	32
Whole milk	27
Artificially sweetened, fruit-flavored yogurt	14

FRUITS

Watermelon	72
Pineapple	66
Cantaloupe	65
Raisins	64
Orange juice	57
Mango	55
Banana	53
Kiwifruit	52
Grapefruit juice	48
Pineapple juice	46
Grapes	43
Orange	43
Apple juice	41
Apple	36
Pear	36
Strawberries	32
Dried apricots	31
Peach	28
Grapefruit	25
Plum	24
Cherries	22

VEGETABLES

Parsnip	97
Baked potato	85
Instant mashed potato	83
French-fried potato	75
Pumpkin	75
Carrot	71

Fresh mashed potato	70
Beet	64
Boiled new potato	62
Fresh corn	59
Sweet potato	54
Yam	51
Green peas	48
Tomato	38

SNACKS AND MISCELLANEOUS

Pretzel	83
Rice cake	82
Vanilla wafers	77
Tortilla chips	74
Corn chips	72
Table sugar (sucrose)	65
Popcorn	55
Potato chips	54
Chocolate	49
Chocolate-covered peanuts	32
Soy milk	31
Peanuts	14

Note: Vegetables not appearing in this table are all low-GI foods.

Source: "International Table of Glycemic Index," as it appears in American Journal of Clinical Nutrition *and* The Glucose Revolution *by Thomas Wolever, MD, PhD*

CHAPTER 13

Pick Your Protein Wisely

Smart cuts can make meat a healthy and tasty part of your weight loss plan

Just because you're on a low-carb diet doesn't mean you have carte blanche to eat all the burgers and tacos you want. Numerous studies show that diets high in saturated fat (the kind found in butter, cheese, and fattier cuts of meat) can lead to heart disease. The key to smart low-carb eating is to replace refined carbs with moderate portions of lean protein foods and unsaturated fats. Though you might end up eating more protein (and meat) than usual, you should still stick to healthy choices, which means choosing mostly poultry, fish, seafood, eggs, some lean cuts of red meat, reduced-fat

The secret to that hi-pro glow.

cheeses, nuts, and maybe a few soy foods. Here are some guidelines to follow.

Order lean cuts. Red meat is rich in iron, zinc, and B vitamins, and it adds variety to your diet. There's no need to swear off it, but try to limit red meats to two or three meals per week. Lean cuts are the smartest choice. If beef is on your menu or shopping list, choose tenderloin, top loin, sirloin, top round, eye of round, tip, or flank steak. For lamb, choose whole leg, loin chop, blade chops, foreshank, or sirloin roast. When choosing pork, look to tenderloin, sirloin, rib chops, lean boneless ham, or Canadian bacon. If you eat veal, any cut except commercially ground will be fairly lean. Game meats such as venison and buffalo are quite lean as well.

Buy the best ground meat. Extra-lean ground beef is the best choice. Try ground turkey for a change, or mix ground beef and ground turkey breast together for juicy hamburgers, meat loaf, meatballs, or chili. If you're a beef purist, mix ground chuck with lean ground sirloin.

Get a higher grade. Reach for meat labeled "select." It will be leaner than meat graded "choice" or "prime." If you can't find select, go for choice.

Make it natural. If you eat cold cuts, try to use those without fillers. Eat only a minimal amount of smoked and cured meats such as ham, bacon, and hot dogs. If you eat these foods, try to have a tomato product at the same meal. It may help protect you from the possible cancer-causing effects of the nitrates and nitrites.

Pick skinny poultry. Most poultry is lean if you avoid the skin. Chicken breasts and legs make good choices. Read labels when buying ground turkey or chicken. Ground turkey breast has the least fat. Seven percent low-fat ground turkey is

DO JUST ONE THING!

Protein plus strength training = healthy aging

Scientists have long believed that we lose muscle as we age because muscle proteins inherently start breaking down faster than we can create them. Not so, say researchers from the University of Texas Medical Branch at Galveston. When they injected 48 men at rest (half, average age 70; half, average age 28) with amino acids (building blocks for muscle), muscle breakdown was similar in both groups. "The actual problem may be that older people's eating and exercise habits deteriorate, and/or they have more trouble using protein from food," says Elena Volpi, MD, PhD, lead researcher and assistant professor of medicine at the University of Southern California in Los Angeles.

Researchers are investigating a number of possible therapies, but for now an exercise program and a wise diet may be the answer. Dr. Volpi recommends that older adults get plenty of protein in the form of eggs, meat, fish, and, if necessary, supplements (ask a registered dietitian), as well as exercise. That alone can help stem the typical muscle loss of 5 lb a decade.

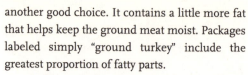

Sneaky Carbs in Seafood

Generally, fish is a healthy choice. But some types of seafood are higher in carbs than others. Here's a ranking of fresh and prepared fish and shellfish to help you make smart choices.

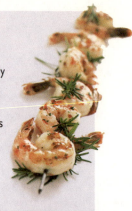

SEAFOOD	CARBS (G)
Deviled crab, 1 cup	32
Breaded, fried scallops, 12	20
Shrimp cocktail, 4 oz (1 jar)	20
Imitation crab, ½ cup	8
Tuna salad (with celery, pickle, onion, egg, and mayonnaise), 1 cup	7
Fish sticks, 3	5
Oysters, raw, ½ cup	4
Scallops, 4 oz	4
Clam, raw, 1	1
Crabmeat, ½ cup	0.5
Lobster meat, 1 cup	0.5
Shrimp, cooked, 1 cup	0

another good choice. It contains a little more fat that helps keep the ground meat moist. Packages labeled simply "ground turkey" include the greatest proportion of fatty parts.

Crack a couple eggs. Most health experts have put eggs back on the menu as a good source of protein. Eggs contain important nutrients in both the yolk and the white. If you're a fan, eat up to six eggs a week. Plus, they're so versatile. Try eggs scrambled, hard-boiled, poached, fried, or made into an omelette, frittata, or egg salad.

Eat more fish. Fish is a terrific source of important healthy fats. Our bodies require two types of dietary fats: omega-6 and omega-3 fatty acids. Research shows that these fats help protect your heart. And they can only be obtained from food because our bodies do not make them. Omega-3 fatty acids are abundant in salmon, tuna, mackerel, herring, sardines, trout, halibut, cod, and bluefish. To boost your heart health, try to eat some type of fish at least twice a week. When you can, choose fresh fish—the flavor beats frozen and canned hands down. But canned tuna and salmon also count as fish meals. If you stock frozen seafood, look for varieties without breading.

Go nuts occasionally. If you don't like fish, look to walnuts and flaxseed for omega-3 fatty acids. Nuts, seeds, nut butters, and nut oils also contain omega-6 fatty acids. Data from a long-term, large-scale research project called the Nurses' Health Study showed that both of these fats can help reduce blood cholesterol levels, blood pressure, and heart disease risk. That's why these essential fatty acids are referred to as healthy fats. The beneficial amount of nuts consumed in the Nurses' Health Study was 5 to 7 oz per week, which translates to a little less than 1 oz of nuts a day. Finally, a snack food that has health benefits!

Go nuts daily. The ancient Romans often served nuts with or after dessert. Hence, the term "from soup to nuts." Take a tip from the ancients, and reap a wealth of health benefits by eating nuts every day, whether for an appetizer, dessert, or on-the-go snack. They contain protein, iron, and other important vitamins and minerals. If you're not a nut lover already, here are some surprising nut facts that might give you a change of heart.

➤ One ounce of almonds (20 to 25 almonds) contains as much calcium as ¼ cup of milk. The same amount also supplies 35% of the Daily Value of vitamin E, plus trace amounts of magnesium, zinc, phosphorus, fiber, and folic acid.

➤ Pecans contain 65 to 70% oil. Most of this oil is the same kind of heart-healthy monounsaturated fat found in olive oil.

➤ Pine nuts have the highest protein content of any nut. Ounce for ounce, pine nuts contain approximately the same amount of protein as beef.

Go nuts at every meal. You can add nuts to almost any dish, be it savory or sweet; they are incredibly versatile. They can be eaten alone as a snack, or sprinkle them on whole grain cereal or yogurt, into bread or cookie batters, into casseroles, on pasta, or over desserts. Pastas and casseroles are typically made with high-glycemic ingredients such as potatoes or breadcrumbs. To lower the glycemic index, add nuts. Pine nuts are terrific with pasta or couscous. Pecans, walnuts, and almonds work well with vegetables and rice dishes. Nuts even work with meats.

Stock up on natural peanut butter. If you like peanut butter, try the unsweetened variety, also called natural peanut butter. Unsweetened peanut butter is made without hydrogenated fats, sugar, or other flavoring agents. It has a more peanutty taste and a lower glycemic index than most commercial varieties, so it won't raise your blood sugar as rapidly.

Give other nut butters a try too. Cashew butter is exceptionally rich tasting and delicious on toast with fruit spread. Creamy macadamia nut butter makes a great sandwich spread. And almond butter is fantastic in sauces. You can use almost any nut butter to make a dip or sauce. Tahini (sesame seed butter) is another good choice for making dips and sauces. These nut butters are sold in most health food stores and some large supermarkets.

What's a Serving of Nuts?

As good as nuts are for you, they're still high in calories, so you should stick to about an ounce a day. See below to find out how many nuts are in 1 oz. Notice that the nuts with fewer calories have more carbohydrates. To get the best balance in low-calorie, low-carb nuts, go for peanuts, pistachios, or pine nuts.

NUT	AMT	CAL	CARBS (G)
Chestnuts	3½	70	15
Cashews	18	163	9
Pistachios	47	160	8
Peanuts	20	166	6
Almonds	22	170	5
Hazelnuts	12	183	5
Pine nuts	155	160	5
Brazil nuts	8	190	4
Macadamias	12	200	4
Pecan halves	15	201	4
Walnut halves	14	185	4

Welcome Back Fat!

The savory flavors you love can *finally* be part of a healthy weight loss diet!

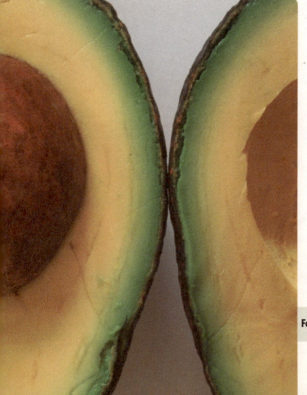

Forbidden no more.

After years of deprivation, fat is back on your plate where it belongs as part of a good-for-you weight loss plan. The emphasis, of course, is on healthy fats, such as those found in olive oil, nuts, and fish. Saturated fat (the kind in cheese, butter, and fatty meats) is still a no-no, since studies show it contributes to heart disease. But if you choose your fats wisely, you can eat your fill and still drop pounds. The following guidelines will keep you on the right track.

Focus on unsaturated fats. Most unsaturated fats come from plant foods rather than animal foods. Both monounsaturated and polyunsaturated fats are considered healthy fats. They are liquid at room temperature as well as in your body. For this reason, they keep cell membranes flexible and fluid. They also reduce your risk of heart disease.

The best choices are monounsaturated: olive oil, canola oil, peanut oil, and avocado. Monounsaturated fats bring down total cholesterol without affecting good HDL levels—a strong asset, given that researchers have detected high cholesterol levels even in teens. Polyunsaturated fats, such as safflower, sesame, and sunflower seeds, corn and soybeans, and other nuts and seeds and their oils, are also good choices. These fats bring down all cholesterol levels. Use mostly liquid oils such as olive and canola for cooking and salads.

Skip the saturated fats. The less saturated fat, the better. Saturated fats, the ones that clog your arteries, are solid at room temperature. Saturated fat is found mostly in animal fats such as butter, full-fat dairy products, meats, and poultry skin, as well as so-called tropical oils such as cocoa butter, coconut oil, palm oil, and palm kernel oil. Try to limit saturated fat to no more than two servings a day (about 2 slices of bacon or 2 tablespoons of cream cheese). Less is even better. Foods high in saturated fat raise cholesterol levels and contribute to heart disease.

Bypass trans fats. Food manufacturers do amazing things to once-healthy liquid oils: They transform them into solid fats. These trans fats are made by heating liquid oils to very high temperatures for 6 to 8 hours, then chemically introducing hydrogen molecules. This results in hydrogenated fats that are less expensive, less perishable, and more spreadable than natural fats. It's a good thing for food manufacturers but not for your body, because hydrogenated oils act more like saturated fat inside you; they tend to raise blood cholesterol levels and increase heart disease risk. Hydrogenated or partially hydrogenated fats are found in most commercially made cookies, pastries, chips, chocolates, crackers, and breads. They're also the key ingredient in stick margarine and the oils used for frying foods in fast-food restaurants. If you can avoid these foods, you'll be close to omitting all trans fats from your diet and thus decreasing your risk of heart disease.

Dip in the tub. If you use margarine instead of butter, buy it in a tub instead of a stick. Tub margarine contains less than half the trans fatty acids of stick margarine. Better yet, look for tub margarines that say "no trans fats" right on the label.

Choose a better butter. If you use butter, limit saturated fat by choosing light butter when you can. Light butter has half the saturated fat and half the calories of regular butter. You can use it in baking, but reduce the amount of liquid in the recipe to compensate for the added water in light butter. For instance, in muffins or pancakes, reduce the amount of milk or juice by about 1/4 cup.

Making smart fat decisions now could affect your cholesterol all the way through menopause and beyond, when women's risk for heart disease increases.

Making smart fat decisions now could affect your cholesterol all the way through menopause and beyond.

Snack Attack!

Can you spot the munchies that fill your stomach without landing on your hips?

Some munchies are easy on your waistline. Others send you directly to the next largest jeans size. But the difference isn't always obvious. Take our quiz, so you'll never be fooled. (Don't peek at the answer before giving yours!)

WHAT'S SKINNIER?
Energy Bar or Chocolate Bar?
ENERGY BAR (but not by much!)

A Balance Gold Rocky Road energy bar (1.76 oz) contains 210 calories, while a Hershey's Milk Chocolate bar (1.55 oz) contains 230 calories. Surprised that the energy bar is almost as high-cal as the candy bar? "Even though the calories are roughly the same, the energy bar has only half as much artery-clogging saturated fat as the candy bar. And the fortified vitamins and minerals in most energy bars do constitute a plus," says Kathryn Miller, RD, nutritionist at The Cooper Aerobics Center in Dallas.

WHAT'S SKINNIER?
High-Fiber Cereal or Doughnuts?
DOUGHNUTS!

Stunned, shocked, and chagrined? So were we. Two Hostess plain doughnuts come in at 300 calories and 16 g of fat. Compare that with the 380 calories and 6 g of fat in 2 cups of Kashi GoLean Crunch! cereal, a popular snack we see lots of dieters munching by the boxful lately. "Portion size is everything," says Karen Miller-Kovach, RD, chief scientist for Weight Watchers in Woodbury, NY. "Limit the calories of the cereal snack by eating only 1 cup for 190 calories versus 2 cups for 380."

WHAT'S SKINNIER?
Granola Bar or Apple?
GRANOLA BAR (sort of)

If calories are your only measure, a 10-oz apple (the size of a baseball on steroids) has about 165 calories, while a Quaker Chewy Chocolate Chip Granola Bar (the size of a Pez dispenser) has 120 calories. But that apple is going to last much longer as a snack than the three-bite granola bar. Plus, the apple has 8 g of fill-you-up fiber; the granola bar has only 1 g of fiber.

WHAT'S SKINNIER?
Tortilla Chips or Veggie Pizza?
AN ENTIRE VEGGIE PIZZA!

A miniature 3.5-oz bag of Doritos Nacho Cheesier!
Tortilla Chips can be extremely deceptive. That little bag holds
only 31 chips, but it delivers 490 calories and
more than 24 g of fat if you eat the whole thing
(which you can easily do). On the other hand, just 3½ minutes at the
microwave makes you an entire Smart Ones Bistro Selections Veggie
Ultimate Pizza for only 400 calories and 5 g of fat.

Admittedly, for most weight-conscious people, the 400 calories in the
pizza might be a little hefty for a snack. But it's certainly fewer calories than
the chips and would probably serve well as a meal, with 5 g of fiber and a dollop
of vitamins and minerals. A word to the calorie-wise: Not all frozen pizzas are low-cal. Read labels so
you know what you're getting.

WHAT'S SKINNIER?
36 Cashews or 12 ½ Cups of Popcorn?
12 ½ CUPS OF POPCORN (by a nose)

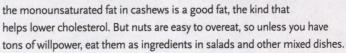

Honestly speaking, most people who eat microwave popcorn do so with
one goal in mind: to wolf down the entire bag in one contented sitting.
But even so, a whole bag of popped Orville Redenbacher's Reden-
Budders Light Movie Theater Butter popcorn (12½ cups' worth)
contains only 312 calories and 6 g of fat. Compare that with 36
cashews (barely two handfuls), which
contain 340 calories and 28 g of fat. True,
the monounsaturated fat in cashews is a good fat, the kind that
helps lower cholesterol. But nuts are easy to overeat, so unless you have
tons of willpower, eat them as ingredients in salads and other mixed dishes.

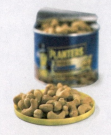

CHAPTER 15

Customize Your Weight Loss Plan

Get the body you've always wanted eating foods you love

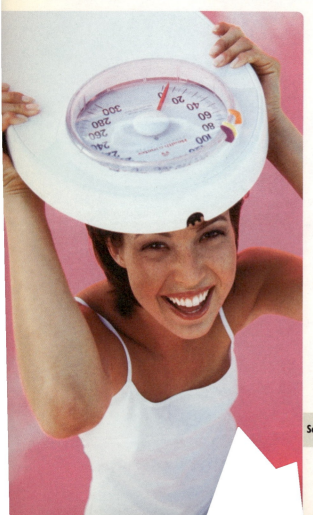

So long, stubborn pounds!

Now that you know how effective and healthy a low-carb diet can be for losing weight, we'll show you how to put it into action. The following plan is tailored to fit your calorie and carbohydrate needs so that you can lose weight—about 1 to 2 lb per week. Start now, and before you know it you'll be dropping those extra pounds and loving your new low-carb lifestyle! Here's how to get started.

Calculate Your Daily Calories

Before you begin, you need to know your daily calorie requirement (how many calories you need to eat to maintain a healthy weight). If you have no idea of your current calorie intake, here's an easy way to find it. First, decide how active you are.

➤ Sedentary means that you have a job or lifestyle that involves mostly sitting, standing, or light walking. You exercise once a week or less.

➤ Active means that your job or lifestyle requires more activity than light walking (such as full-time housecleaning or construction work), or you get 45 to 60 minutes of aerobic exercise three times a week.

➤ Very active means that you get aerobic exercise for at least 45 to 60 minutes four or more times a week.

Choose the description that best fits your current lifestyle, then find your activity factor from the table below.

YOUR ACTIVITY FACTOR

IF YOU ARE A . . .	FACTOR IS . . .
Sedentary woman	12
Sedentary man	14
Active woman	15
Active man	17
Very active woman	18
Very active man	20

Multiply your activity factor by your current weight in pounds. The resulting number is the approximate number of calories you currently need to maintain your weight. The math looks like this: *activity factor x weight in pounds = current calorie needs*

Here's an example for an active woman who weighs 150 lb: 15 x 150 = 2,250

ADJUST YOUR INTAKE

Rather than choosing a goal weight, simply reduce your current calorie intake by 500 to 1,000 calories a day. (Never go below 1,500 calories a day unless under the supervision of a doctor.) This will lead to safe, effective weight loss of 1 to 2 lb per week. For instance, if you currently take in 2,300 to 2,500 calories a day, try reducing your daily intake to 1,800 to 2,000 calories. This will be your new daily calorie level.

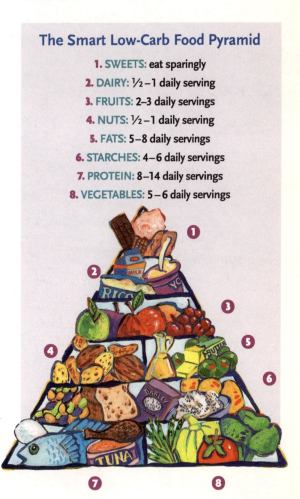

The Smart Low-Carb Food Pyramid

1. SWEETS: eat sparingly
2. DAIRY: ½–1 daily serving
3. FRUITS: 2–3 daily servings
4. NUTS: ½–1 daily serving
5. FATS: 5–8 daily servings
6. STARCHES: 4–6 daily servings
7. PROTEIN: 8–14 daily servings
8. VEGETABLES: 5–6 daily servings

Count Up Your Carbs

Carbohydrates in the average diet supply 50 to 60% of total calories. Based on your calorie level that you just calculated, check the table at right to find out the approximate grams of carbohydrates in your diet. You might be surprised by how many carbohydrates you actually eat now. This table is based upon 55% of calories from carbohydrates, the average percentage consumed by most Americans. If your diet is more heavily weighted in carbohydrates, the figures may be on the low side.

DAILY CALORIES	CARBS (G)
1,800	248
2,000	275
2,400	330
2,800	385
3,000	413

SHOOT FOR 125 G

Most people who now consume a low-fat, high-carbohydrate diet (the standard American weight loss diet) will likely lose weight by cutting carbohydrates down to 125 g and replacing

---

DO JUST ONE THING!

Your Perfect Weight Loss Plan

Personalizing your diet has never been easier. Simply choose the calorie level that is right for you, then eat from the food groups listed below. This will automatically make you cut back on your carbs yet make sure you get enough of the right foods. To choose your calorie level, see p. 105.

CALORIES	1,500–1,800			1,800–2,200		
Food Group	Servings	Cal	Carb (g)	Servings	Cal	Carb (g)
Protein	9	495	0	14	890	0
Fat	6	270	0	8	360	0
Nuts	1	200	4	1	200	4
Vegetables	5	125	25	5	125	25
Starches	4	320	60	4	320	60
Fruits	2	120	30	2	120	30
Dairy	0.5	45	6	0.5	45	6
Total		1,575	125		2,060	125

them with protein and fats. To do that, follow "Your Perfect Weight Loss Plan" at left. Simply eat the daily number of food servings listed under that plan. For example, if you follow the 125-g plan at 1,800 to 2,200 calories, you should eat 14 servings of protein foods, 8 servings of fats, 1 serving of nuts, 5 servings of veggies, 4 servings of starches, 2 servings of fruit, and $^{1}/_{2}$ serving of milk-based foods.

SHAVE SATURATED FAT

Notice that on each plan, as the servings of carbohydrate foods (such as starch, fruit, and milk) go down, the servings of protein foods and fat foods go up. Be sure to choose the healthiest protein and fat foods you can find. For protein, that means fish, eggs, poultry, and occasionally lean cuts of beef, pork, and lamb. For fats, focus on mono- and polyunsaturated fats such as olive oil, canola oil, nut oils, and avocados, instead of butter, bacon, and salt pork. These healthier choices will help minimize your intake of saturated fat, thereby helping to prevent heart disease. Try to eat no more than two servings of saturated fat a day. Less is even better.

WATCH FOR HIDDEN CARBS

Fats and protein foods have no carbohydrate, but the other food groups contain varying amounts of carbohydrate. Generally, one serving of vegetables contains 5 g of carbs, one serving of milk contains 12 g, and one serving of starch or fruit contains 15 g. Because these food groups all contain carbohydrate, you can interchange them now and then (at right).

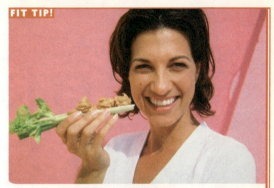

FIT TIP!

Prepare for the snack attack
Stash low-carb snacks in your kitchen, desk, car, or tote. Nuts and cheeses are really satisfying in a pinch. Pine nuts, in particular, are high in protein and very filling. Keep a jar of nut butter or a package of cream cheese on hand to spread on ribs of celery for a snack. Or snack on string cheese or other hard cheeses.

MAKE SMART SUBSTITUTIONS

If there are certain foods unavailable to you on a particular day, or if you don't care to eat the ones that are, you can substitute foods from other groups. See the suggested substitutions below. The numbers of carbohydrate grams are roughly equivalent.

FOOD GROUP	SUGGESTED SUBSTITUTION
starch, 1 serving	milk, $^{1}/_{2}$ serving + fruit, $^{1}/_{2}$ serving
milk, 1 serving	starch, 1 serving
fruit, $^{1}/_{2}$ serving	milk, $^{1}/_{2}$ serving + vegetable, 1 serving
nuts, 1 serving	vegetable, 1 serving + fat, 2 servings
vegetable, 1 serving	fruit, $^{1}/_{2}$ serving

part 5

real meals you'll love

110   ## 7 Days to a Slimmer You
An easy-to-follow meal plan to start you
on the road to low-carb success

122   ## Start the Day the Smart Low-Carb Way
These quick and yummy morning meals will get
your day—and diet—started off in the right direction

128   ## Real Power Lunches
Try these easy-to-make, high-protein dishes
for fast and slimming midday meals

134   ## Savory Dinners
One bite of these filling, flavorful dishes, and
you'll never look at low-carb the same way again

145   ## Just Desserts
These yummy treats prove that low-carb dieters
can have their cake (and pudding and cookies)
and their waistline too

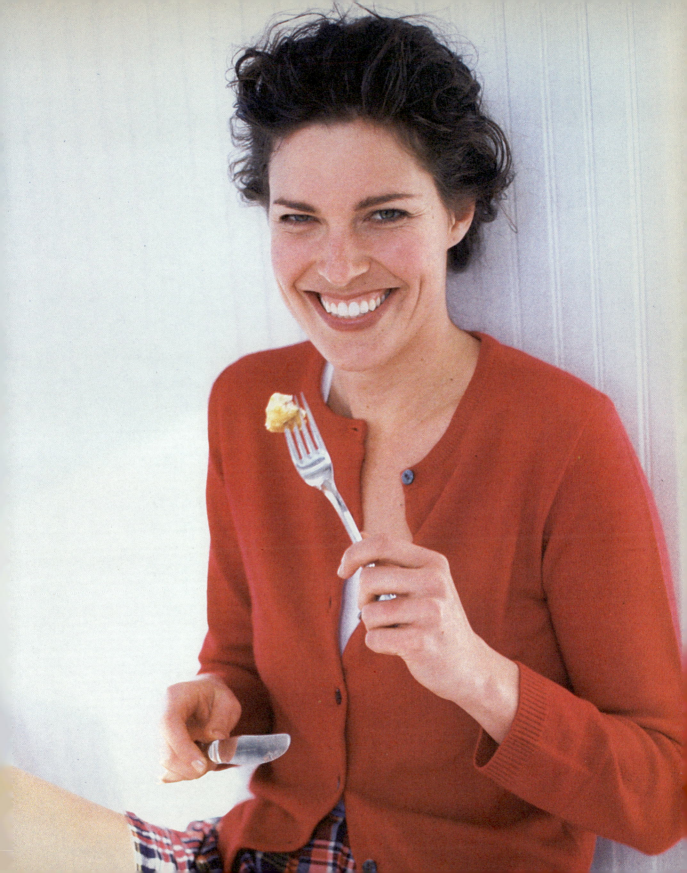

7 Days to a Slimmer You

An easy-to-follow meal plan to start you
on the road to low-carb success

Now you're really ready to get a taste of smart low-carb eating. We took the best recipes (and a few other common foods) and organized them into a variety of great-tasting, balanced meals. Each daily menu includes three main meals and three snacks. Just one look, and you'll see that losing weight does not mean depriving yourself.

Each of these menus contains approximately 125 g of carbohydrate per day (the 125-g plan outlined on p. 106). Beverages aren't included here. They're up to you. Remember that water, tea, coffee, seltzer, and club soda are all calorie-free and carbohydrate-free.

These meals offer a great starting place for weight loss. Adjust the foods to fit your personal likes and dislikes. And once you start eating the smart low-carb way, experiment by creating your own menus. In just 7 days, you should look—and feel—a whole lot better!

**Time for those
new jeans!**

Day 1

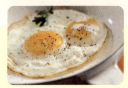

MENU	CALORIE LEVELS	
	1,500–1,800	**1,800–2,200**
Breakfast		
Fried Eggs with Vinegar (p. 122)	1 serving	1 serving
Fat-free milk	½ cup	½ cup
Apple juice	½ cup	½ cup
Whole grain bread	1 slice	1 slice
Butter	1 tsp	1 tsp
Snack		
Nectarine or pear	1	1
Lunch		
Grilled chicken tenders brushed	4 oz	5 oz
with Italian dressing	1 tsp	1 Tbsp
Red leaf lettuce	1 cup	1 cup
Carrot, shredded	¼ cup	¼ cup
Cucumber, sliced	½ cup	½ cup
Italian dressing	2 tsp	2 Tbsp
Snack		
Walnuts	1 oz	1 oz
Dinner		
London broil	4 oz	5 oz
Spanish-Style Green Beans (p. 134)	1 serving	1 serving
Couscous	½ cup	½ cup
Snack		
Orange-Walnut Biscotti (p. 146)	2	2
TOTAL CALORIES (APPROX)	**1,640**	**1,880**
TOTAL CARBS (G)	**125**	**125**

Day 2

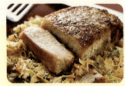

MENU	CALORIE LEVELS	
	1,500–1,800	**1,800–2,200**
Breakfast		
Cherry Cream of Rye Cereal (p. 123)	1 serving	1 serving
Fat-free milk	½ cup	½ cup
Turkey sausage	1 oz	1 oz
Snack		
Apple	1	1
Lunch		
Tuna	3 oz	4 oz
Celery, chopped	¼ cup	¼ cup
Onion, chopped	¼ cup	¼ cup
Mayonnaise, reduced-fat	2 Tbsp	¼ cup
Green olives	10 small	10 small
Green leaf lettuce, torn	1 cup	1 cup
Sourdough bread	1 slice	1 slice
Snack		
Pecans	1 oz	1 oz
Dinner		
Pork Chops Baked with Cabbage and Cream (p. 135)	1 serving	1 serving
Steamed butternut squash	½ cup	½ cup
Snack		
Pumpernickel bread	1 slice	slice
Swiss cheese, reduced-fat	1 oz	2 oz
Butter	1 tsp	2 tsp
TOTAL CALORIES (APPROX)	1,670	1,960
TOTAL CARBS (G)	127	127

Day 3

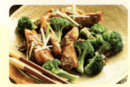

MENU	CALORIE LEVELS	
	1,500–1,800	1,800–2,200
Breakfast		
Scrambled egg	1	2
Orange juice	¹/₂ cup	¹/₂ cup
Rye toast	1 slice	1 slice
Butter	1 tsp	2 tsp
Fat-free milk	¹/₂ cup	¹/₂ cup
Snack		
Kiwifruit	1	1
Lunch		
Salad consisting of:		
Lentils, cooked	¹/₂ cup	¹/₂ cup
Turkey breast, cooked and cubed	3 oz	4 oz
Carrot, sliced	¹/₂ cup	¹/₂ cup
Peppers, chopped	¹/₂ cup	¹/₂ cup
Peas, cooked	¹/₄ cup	¹/₄ cup
Olive oil	2 tsp	1 Tbsp
Cheddar cheese	¹/₂ oz	¹/₂ oz
Snack		
Brazil nuts	1 oz	1 oz
Dinner		
Stir-Fried Chicken and Broccoli (p. 136)	1 serving (4 oz chicken)	1 serving (5 oz chicken)
Snack		
Pecan Muffins (p. 124)	1	1
Butter	1 tsp	2 tsp
TOTAL CALORIES (APPROX)	1,590	1,960
TOTAL CARBS (G)	123	123

Day 4

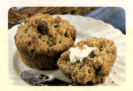

MENU	CALORIE LEVELS	
	1,500–1,800	1,800–2,200
Breakfast		
Pecan Muffins (p. 124)	1	1
Cottage cheese	2 Tbsp	6 Tbsp
Peach	1	1
Fat-free milk	½ cup	½ cup
Snack		
Grapefruit	½	½
Lunch		
Sandwich of rice cakes (2) topped with:		
Sardines, boneless, skinless	4 oz	5 oz
Cream cheese	2 Tbsp	2 Tbsp
Tomato	2 slices	2 slices
Zucchini, sticks	½ cup	½ cup
Snack		
Almonds	1 oz	1 oz
Dinner		
Lamb chop, baked with	4 oz	5 oz
garlic powder	⅛ tsp	⅛ tsp
Mint leaves, chopped	2 tsp	1 Tbsp
Barley, cooked	½ cup	½ cup
Stewed tomatoes	1 cup	1 cup
Green beans, sautéed in	½ cup	½ cup
olive oil	2 tsp	3 tsp
Snack		
Whole wheat bread	1 slice	1 slice
Butter	1 tsp	2 tsp
Chicken, sliced	1 oz	2 oz
TOTAL CALORIES (APPROX)	1,700	1,950
TOTAL CARBS (G)	122	122

Day 5

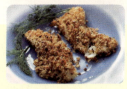

MENU	CALORIE LEVELS	
	1,500–1,800	**1,800–2,200**
Breakfast		
Sweet potato, cooked and topped	½ cup	½ cup
with walnut oil or canola oil	½ tsp	1 tsp
Walnuts, chopped	1 oz	1 oz
Coconut, shredded	1 Tbsp	2 Tbsp
Pineapple, crushed	¼ cup	¼ cup
Chicken breast, cooked	——	2 oz
Fat-free milk	½ cup	½ cup
Snack		
Pear	½	½
Lunch		
Salad of spinach and:	2 cups	2 cups
Chickpeas	½ cup	½ cup
Egg, hard-boiled	1	2
Artichoke hearts	½ cup	½ cup
Olive oil	2 tsp	3 tsp
Lemon juice	1 Tbsp	1 Tbsp
Whole wheat pita	½	½
Snack		
Monterey Jack cheese	2 oz	2 oz
Dinner		
Breaded Baked Cod with Tartar Sauce (p. 137)	1 serving	1 serving
Red cabbage,	½ cup	½ cup
sautéed in sesame oil	1 tsp	2 tsp
Yellow squash, steamed	½ cup	½ cup
Butter	1 tsp	1 tsp
Cantaloupe Sorbet (p. 145)	1 serving	1 serving
Snack		
Popcorn, air-popped	3 cups	3 cups
Butter	1 tsp	2 tsp
Monterey Jack cheese	2 oz	2 oz
TOTAL CALORIES (APPROX)	**1,640**	**1,980**
TOTAL CARBS (G)	**124**	**124**

Day 6

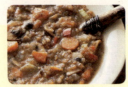

MENU	CALORIE LEVELS	
	1,500–1,800	1,800–2,200
Breakfast		
Cottage cheese	¼ cup	½ cup
Blueberries	¾ cup	¾ cup
Cinnamon	Pinch	Pinch
Bacon, nitrate-free, cooked	1 slice	2 slices
Snack		
Grapes, red	15 small	15 small
Lunch		
Hamburger, lean	4 oz	5 oz
Hamburger bun, whole wheat	½	½
Leaf lettuce	1 leaf	1 leaf
Tomato	1 slice	1 slice
Onion	1 slice	1 slice
Mustard	1 tsp	1 tsp
Mayonnaise, reduced-fat	2 tsp	3 tsp
French fries	10 small	10 small
Green olives	——	5 small
Snack		
Hazelnuts	1 oz	1 oz
Cheddar cheese, reduced-fat	——	1½ oz
Dinner		
Mushroom and Kasha Soup (p. 138)	1 serving	1 serving
Turkey breast, cooked	4 oz	5 oz
Carrots, baby, cooked	½ cup	½ cup
Peas, cooked	¼ cup	¼ cup
Olive oil	1 tsp	2 tsp
Snack		
Peanut Butter Cookies (p. 147)	1	1
Fat-free milk	½ cup	½ cup
TOTAL CALORIES (APPROX)	1,570	1,890
TOTAL CARBS (G)	125	125

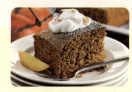

Day 7

MENU	CALORIE LEVELS	
	1,500–1,800	**1,800–2,200**
Breakfast		
Bran cereal, flaked	½ cup	½ cup
Fat-free milk	½ cup	½ cup
Banana	½	½
Cottage cheese	½ cup	½ cup
Snack		
Cherries, large	10	10
Protein bar (16 g pro, 2 g carb)	——	¾ bar
Lunch		
Sausage, Egg, and Vegetable Casserole (p. 129)	1 serving	1 serving
Spinach, steamed	½ cup	½ cup
Whole wheat bread	1 slice	1 slice
Snack		
Almonds	1 oz	1 oz
Swiss cheese, reduced-fat	——	2 oz
Dinner		
Scallops in Tarragon Cream (p. 139)	1 serving	1 serving
Asparagus, steamed	½ cup	½ cup
Tomato, broiled	1 large	1 large
Brown rice, cooked	½ cup	½ cup
Butter	——	1 tsp
Snack		
Gingerbread Cake with Peach Whipped Cream (p. 148)	1 serving	1 serving
TOTAL CALORIES (APPROX)	**1,530**	**1,950**
TOTAL CARBS (G)	**128**	**128**

Just the FAQs

All your low-carb questions (and some you never thought to ask!) answered

Solid research and clinical observations have convinced us that smart low-carb eating is the way to go for losing weight and staying healthy. But you may have some concerns based on warnings that have circulated regarding low-carb diets. Here are the answers to health questions that have been raised by doctors, nutritionists, and other skeptics of lower-carbohydrate diets.

Q: Will following this diet give me bad breath?

A: No. The dreaded "ketone breath" associated with other low-carbohydrate diets is not a problem on this plan because the carbohydrates are not as restricted. Ketones are chemicals produced when your body runs out of stored glycogen (blood sugar) and starts burning only fat for energy. Ketones are used as fuel or expelled from the body through your breath or urination. Ketosis, the term for the process, occurs during fasting, pregnancy, and on diets very low in carbs. We advocate a smart lower-carbohydrate approach avoiding refined carbs, but not the severe carbohydrate restriction that triggers ketosis.

Q: Will eating more protein and fewer carbohydrates damage my kidneys?

A: Probably not. If you've never had a kidney problem, you probably don't need to worry about the warnings that eating more protein and fewer carbohydrates will wear out your kidneys. There is no research confirming this potential danger, even in people who consume three times the recommended amount of protein. Do pay attention to the warning if you already have kidney disease. A higher protein intake may be dangerous if your kidneys are not functioning properly. If you're unsure whether your kidneys are healthy, consult your doctor before changing your diet.

Q: Won't eating more fat raise my cholesterol and triglycerides and increase my risk of heart disease?

A: Quite the opposite. We have all been brainwashed into believing that eating foods with any type of fat will cause elevated cholesterol in everyone who eats them. However, saturated fat is the real culprit in increased heart disease risk. We've talked with several people who regularly eat foods high in mono- and polyunsaturated fats while reducing their carbohydrate intake, and their total cholesterol has actually come down. Most people who eat fewer carbohydrates find that their triglyceride levels go down, and their good HDL cholesterol goes up. The bottom line is that a reduced-carbohydrate eating plan may help reduce your risk of heart disease because it brings down your insulin levels and your triglycerides.

Q: Does restricting carbohydrates reduce energy and cause fatigue?

A: Not likely. Some folks experience fatigue during the first 1 to 3 days. This may be the result of withdrawal from refined sugar, refined wheat, or other foods that the body may have been accustomed to digesting frequently. Yes, energy production is the main function of carbohydrates. However, you will get plenty of energy from the carbohydrates you do include on this plan as well as from the proteins and fats. Fatigue and energy loss are often signs of low blood sugar, and the smart low-carb approach keeps your blood sugar levels stable.

Q: Can a reduced-carbohydrate/ higher-protein plan lead to osteoporosis?

A: This is one warning to keep in mind, though you should be fine if you follow the plan's calcium and vegetable recommendations. Increased protein makes the blood more acidic. The body responds by releasing calcium from the bones to bring the pH to a more alkaline level. However, if you eat lots of vegetables, you will minimize this problem because vegetables make the body more alkaline. Too little protein can also be harmful to the skeleton. To safeguard against osteoporosis, the eating plan is high in calcium-rich foods such as cheese, dark green leafy vegetables, almonds, Brazil nuts, salmon, sardines, and calcium-fortified soy products. Plus, we recommend a wide variety of foods and a daily multivitamin.

Q: I've heard that there is a link between meat and cancer. Is this true?

A: Just keep this motto in mind: Moderation in all things. Eating lots of vegetables and some fruits will supply important antioxidants that help protect us from cancer. Also, remember that the body has a wonderful built-in detoxification system in the liver. Eating a wide variety of whole foods as this plan encourages will supply nutrients that support liver function. Cruciferous vegetables such as broccoli, cauliflower, brussels sprouts, kale, and cabbage are particularly helpful. And keep in mind that our plan recommends eating more protein, but not necessarily more meat. If you prefer not to get your protein from meat, there are recipes and suggestions for getting protein from beans, nuts, and other nonanimal sources.

Q: Will eating more protein increase my risk of heart disease?

A: On the contrary; the science says otherwise. A study at the Harvard School of Public Health looked at 80,082 women ages 34 to 59 without any previous indication of heart disease. When all other risks for heart disease were controlled for, and irrespective of whether the women were on high- or low-fat diets, the results showed that both animal and vegetable proteins contributed to lower risk of heart disease. Researchers concluded that replacing refined carbohydrates with protein may reduce heart disease risk.

Create a Low-Carb Kitchen
Make healthy eating a snap by stocking up on these smart low-carb staples

Here's a list of the low-carb foods you should keep on hand to whip up delicious, diet-friendly meals—a big plus on harried work nights when KFC is calling your name. Some of the refrigerator items such as parsley and lemons may not last as long as other foods, but they have so many uses and are so inexpensive, it's wise to consider them staples. In addition to the foods below, be sure to stock the foods that your family likes best, even some of the higher-carbohydrate ones. If eating high-carb foods now and then helps you stick to your overall eating plan, then it's worth keeping them around. Smart tip: Make several photocopies of this list, and tack them to your fridge, or keep them in a drawer. Each one is a ready-made shopping list that you can tailor to your needs before heading to the store.

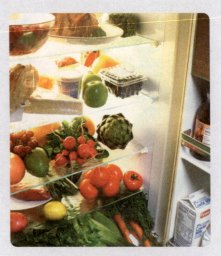

Cool, Dry Place
- Bananas
- Garlic
- Melon (cantaloupe, honeydew, watermelon)
- Onions
- Oranges
- Plums
- Sweet potatoes
- Winter squash

Refrigerator/Freezer
- Butter (preferably light)
- Cheese (Cheddar, mozzarella, Parmesan, Monterey Jack, cream cheese—preferably reduced-fat)
- Eggs
- Half-and-half
- Milk (1%)
- Orange juice
- Sour cream (reduced-fat)
- Yogurt (low-fat, plain)
- Apples
- Bell peppers
- Broccoli
- Cabbage (green or red)
- Carrots
- Cauliflower
- Celery
- Cucumbers
- Eggplant
- Fresh greens
- Grapefruit
- Grapes
- Lemons
- Mushrooms
- Parsley
- Raisins
- Scallions
- Squash (yellow squash, zucchini)
- Nuts (walnuts, pecans, almonds, pine nuts, pistachios, macadamias)
- Seeds (sunflower, sesame)

Freezer

Tortillas (corn and whole wheat)	Veggie burgers
Whole wheat bread	Bacon (pork or turkey)
Broccoli	Beef (lean ground, tenderloin, various steaks)
Corn	Chicken (skinless, boneless breasts and bone-in parts)
Green beans	Lamb (ground, chops)
Peas	Pork (chops and tenderloin)
Spinach	Sausage (pork or turkey)
Salmon	Turkey (cutlets, tenderloin, ground breast)
Shrimp	Frozen fruit (no sugar added)
	Unsweetened coconut

Pantry

Apple juice (or cider in the fridge)	Hot-pepper sauce
Dried apricots	Low-sugar marinara sauce
Dried mushrooms	Mayonnaise (no added sugar)
Canned broth (chicken and beef)	Mustard
Canned chopped clams	Pesto
Canned fish (tuna, salmon, sardines, anchovies, trout fillets)	Salt
Canned fruit in fruit juice	Vinegar (cider, white wine, red wine, balsamic)
Canned mild green chiles	Soy sauce
Canned tomato products (whole, crushed, sauce, juice)	Worcestershire sauce
Dry or canned beans (black, white, pinto, red kidney, chickpeas, brown lentils)	Brown sugar (or brown sugar substitute)
Oats	Splenda
Oat flour	Stevia
Soy flour	All-fruit spread (various flavors)
Whole wheat couscous	Maple syrup (low-calorie)
Whole wheat flour	Peanuts (unsalted, dry-roasted) and nuts
Whole wheat pasta	Peanut butter, natural (and other natural nut butters)
Whole wheat pastry flour	Canola oil
Brown rice	Olive oil
Pearl barley	Sesame oil
Quinoa	Olives
	Roasted peppers
	Tea (regular and herbal)
	Unsweetened cocoa powder
	Whole grain crackers

CHAPTER 17

Start the Day the Smart Low-Carb Way

These quick and yummy morning meals will get your day—and diet—started off in the right direction

Fried Eggs with Vinegar

206 CAL, 1 G CARB

    2   Tbsp butter
    8   lg eggs
    1   tsp salt
   ¼   tsp ground black pepper
   ⅛   tsp dried marjoram or basil
    4   tsp red wine vinegar
    1   tsp chopped parsley (optional)

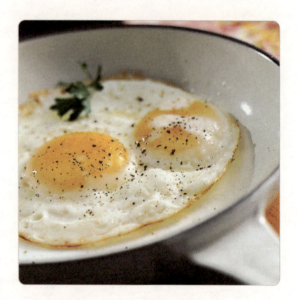

1. Melt 1 tablespoon of the butter in a large non-stick skillet over medium-low heat. Add the eggs, and sprinkle with the salt, pepper, and marjoram (work in batches if necessary). Cover, and cook until the whites are set and the yolks are almost set, 3 to 5 minutes. (For steam-basted eggs, add 1 teaspoon of water to the skillet, and cover with a lid.)

2. Remove to plates. Place the skillet over low heat, and add the remaining 1 tablespoon butter.

Cook until the butter turns light brown, 1 to 2 minutes. Add the vinegar. Pour the vinegar mixture over the eggs. Sprinkle with the parsley (if using). Serve hot. **Makes 4 servings**

PER SERVING: 206 cal, 13 g pro, 1 g carb, 16 g fat, 7 g sat. fat, 440 mg chol, 0 g fiber, 764 mg sodium
DIET EXCHANGES: 0 milk, 0 vegetable, 0 fruit, 0 bread, 2 meat, 2½ fat

Cherry Cream of Rye Cereal

208 CAL, 45 G CARB

- 1¼ c water
- 1¼ c apple cider
- ¼ tsp salt
- 1 c cream of rye cereal
- 1¼ Tbsp cherry fruit spread
- ⅛ tsp ground nutmeg
- ⅛ tsp ground cardamom
- 1½ Tbsp chopped hazelnuts (optional)

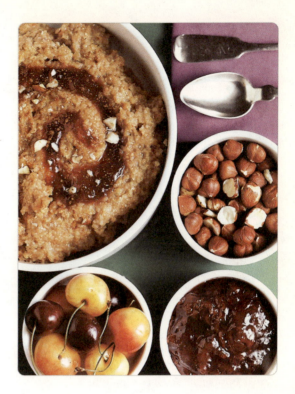

1. Combine the water, cider, and salt in a saucepan, and bring to a boil over medium heat. Stir in the cereal, and reduce the heat to low. Cook, uncovered, until thick, stirring occasionally, 3 to 5 minutes. Remove from the heat, and stir in the fruit spread.

   2. Spoon into bowls, and sprinkle with the nutmeg, cardamom, and hazelnuts (if using). Serve hot. **Makes 4 servings (3 cups)**

PER SERVING: 208 cal, 4 g pro, 45 g carb, 1 g fat, 0 g sat. fat, 0 mg chol, 6 g fiber, 168 mg sodium

DIET EXCHANGES: 0 milk, 0 vegetable, 1 fruit, 2 bread, 0 meat, 0 fat

FIT TIP!

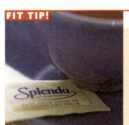

Substitute your sugar

Sweet alternatives can spare your waistline. Some of these recipes use Splenda, a newly available type of sweetener. The primary ingredient in Splenda is sucralose, a sugar substitute processed from real sugar that has been modified so that it isn't absorbed by the body. Sucralose is calorie-free and does not effect blood sugar levels. It measures cup for cup like sugar and performs like sugar in recipes. Another sugar alternative is stevia, an herb that is the only truly all-natural sugar substitute. You can find it in the herbal section of health food stores or large supermarkets in the form of a white powder or liquid. Go easy, since ⅛ teaspoon of liquid stevia is equivalent to ½ cup of sugar.

Pecan Muffins

218 CAL, 20 G CARB

1½	c whole grain pastry flour
¼	c soy flour
2½	tsp baking powder
½	tsp salt
½	tsp ground nutmeg
½	c toasted pecans, chopped
½	c vegetable oil
½	c apricot or peach fruit spread
2	lg eggs, lightly beaten
1½	tsp vanilla extract
⅛	tsp liquid stevia

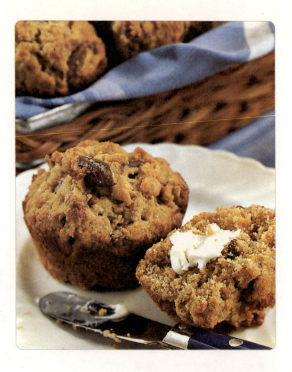

1. Place a rack in the middle position in the oven, and preheat the oven to 375°F. Coat a 12-cup muffin pan with cooking spray, or line it with paper cups.

2. In a large bowl, whisk together the flours, baking powder, salt, nutmeg, and pecans.

3. In a small bowl, combine the oil, fruit spread, eggs, vanilla extract, and stevia. Add to the flour mixture, and stir just until the dry ingredients are moistened.

4. Spoon into the prepared muffin cups until three-quarter full. Bake until a toothpick inserted in the center of a muffin comes out clean, 12 to 14 minutes. Serve warm. **Makes 12**

PER MUFFIN: 218 cal, 4 g pro, 20 g carb, 12 g fat, 1 g sat. fat, 35 mg chol, 3 g fiber, 193 mg sodium

DIET EXCHANGES: 0 milk, 0 vegetable, 0 fruit, 1 bread, ½ meat, 2½ fat

Whole Grain Crepes with Banana and Kiwifruit

215 CAL, 34 G CARB

Crepes
1	c whole grain pastry flour
¼	tsp salt
1	egg
1	c + 3 Tbsp unsweetened soy milk or whole milk
1½	tsp vanilla extract
2	tsp butter
1–2	Tbsp water (optional)

Filling
½	c plain yogurt
1	banana, cut into 24 diagonal slices
2	kiwifruit, peeled, cut in half lengthwise, and sliced
2	tsp lime juice (optional)
½	tsp ground cinnamon

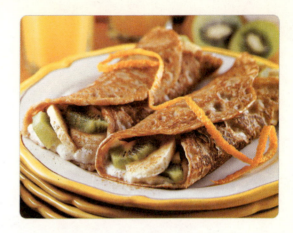

1. *To make the crepes:* In a large bowl, combine the flour and salt.

2. In a small bowl, beat the egg, then stir in the milk and vanilla extract. Pour into the flour, and mix well.

3. Melt ½ teaspoon of the butter in an 8" nonstick skillet over medium heat. Pour 3 tablespoons of batter into the skillet, and tilt the skillet to coat the bottom in a thin layer (if the batter seems too thick, add 1 to 2 tablespoons of water). Cook the first side until nicely browned, about 2 minutes. Using a spatula, turn the crepe, and cook the second side for 1 to 2 minutes (the second side will look spotty).

4. Slide the crepe onto a plate, and cover with foil to keep warm. Continue making crepes in the same fashion, rebuttering the pan after every second crepe, until all the butter and batter are used.

5. *To make the filling and assemble:* Place a crepe on a serving plate, attractive side down, and spread with 1 tablespoon of the yogurt. Arrange 2 banana slices and a quarter of a kiwifruit in strips one-third of the way from one edge. Sprinkle with ¼ teaspoon of the lime juice (if using) and a pinch of the cinnamon, and roll up. Continue assembling the remaining crepes in the same fashion. **Makes 4 servings (eight 6" to 7" crepes)**

PER SERVING: 215 cal, 8 g pro, 34 g carb, 6 g fat, 3 g sat. fat, 62 mg chol, 6 g fiber, 198 mg sodium

DIET EXCHANGES: ½ milk, 0 vegetable, 1 fruit, 1 bread, 0 meat, 1 fat

Baked Apples

176 CAL, 27 G CARB

- 4 Rome apples
- 5 lg pitted prunes or dried apricots, chopped
- 2 Tbsp pine nuts
- 2 tsp apricot or other all-fruit spread (optional)
- $\frac{1}{2}$ tsp pumpkin pie spice
- 4 tsp butter, cut into 4 equal pieces
- $\frac{3}{4}$ c apple cider or water
- $\frac{1}{4}$ c plain yogurt

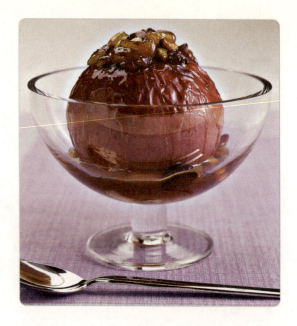

1. Preheat the oven to 375°F.

2. Core the apples to within $\frac{1}{2}$" of their bottoms. Using a paring knife, remove a $\frac{1}{2}$"-wide strip around the top edges. If necessary, trim a thin slice from each bottom so the apples sit flat.

3. In a small bowl, combine the prunes, nuts, all-fruit spread (if using), and pumpkin pie spice. Spoon into the apple cavities, and place the apples in a shallow baking dish.

4. Slip a piece of butter into each cavity, and pour the cider over the apples (the liquid should be $\frac{1}{4}$" to $\frac{1}{2}$" deep in the dish).

5. Bake, uncovered, basting with the pan juices occasionally (add a little hot water if necessary), until the apples are tender when pierced with a fork, 30 to 45 minutes. Place on plates, and spoon the pan juices over them. Serve hot, warm, or at room temperature topped with a dollop of the yogurt. **Makes 4 servings**

PER SERVING: 176 cal, 2 g pro, 27 g carb, 7 g fat, 3 g sat. fat, 12 mg chol, 5 g fiber, 54 mg sodium

DIET EXCHANGES: $\frac{1}{2}$ milk, 0 vegetable, 1$\frac{1}{2}$ fruit, 0 bread, 0 meat, 1 fat

Puffy Frittata with Ham and Green Pepper

290 CAL, 8 G CARB

- 2 Tbsp butter
- 1 sm onion, chopped
- 1 green bell pepper, chopped
- ½ tsp salt
- ½ tsp black pepper
- 8 slices (6 oz total) ham, chopped
- 8 lg eggs, at room temperature
- ¼ c water
- ½ c shredded Cheddar cheese (optional)

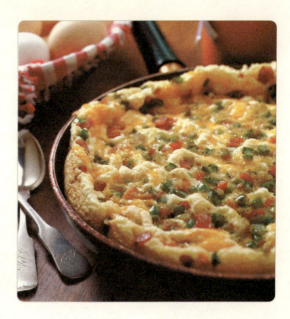

1. Preheat the oven to 250°F.

2. Melt 1 tablespoon of the butter in a large nonstick skillet over low heat. Add the onion, bell pepper, ¼ teaspoon of the salt, and ¼ teaspoon of the pepper. Cook, stirring occasionally, until crisp-tender, 3 to 4 minutes. Stir in the ham, and cook for 1 minute, stirring occasionally. Transfer to a plate.

3. Separate the eggs, placing the yolks in a medium-size bowl and the whites in a large bowl. Lightly beat the yolks with the water, the remaining ¼ teaspoon salt, and the remaining ¼ teaspoon pepper. Beat the egg whites until they form stiff, but not dry, peaks. Fold the yolks into the whites.

4. Melt the remaining 1 tablespoon butter in the skillet over low heat. Pour in the eggs, and spread them evenly with a rubber spatula. Scatter the ham mixture and cheese (if using) over the top, cover, and cook until the eggs are set, 25 to 30 minutes.

5. Slide the frittata onto a plate, and serve immediately (puffiness will subside in 5 to 7 minutes). **Makes 4 servings**

PER SERVING: 290 cal, 22 g pro, 8 g carb, 19 g fat, 5 g sat. fat, 448 mg chol, 2 g fiber, 467 mg sodium

DIET EXCHANGES: 0 milk, 1½ vegetable, 0 fruit, 0 bread, 3 meat, 2 fat

CHAPTER 18

Real Power Lunches

Try these easy-to-make, high-protein dishes for fast and slimming midday meals

Roast Beef Sandwich with Mustard-Horseradish Mayonnaise

349 CAL, 22 G CARB

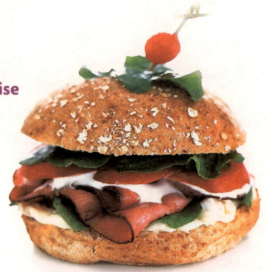

3	Tbsp mayonnaise
2	tsp Dijon mustard
2	tsp prepared horseradish
8	slices light whole wheat bread
12	spinach or lettuce leaves
1/2	cucumber, peeled and thinly sliced
12	slices roast beef (3/4 lb)
1/2	tsp salt
1/4	tsp ground black pepper

In a small bowl, combine the mayonnaise, mustard, and horseradish. Spread over the bread, and cover 4 of the slices with the spinach. Arrange the cucumber and beef over the spinach. Season with the salt and pepper. Top with the remaining bread, and cut in half. **Makes 4 servings**

PER SERVING: 349 cal, 30 g pro, 22 g carb, 17 g fat, 4 g sat. fat, 73 mg chol, 7 g fiber, 734 mg sodium

DIET EXCHANGES: 0 milk, 1/2 vegetable, 0 fruit, 1 1/2 bread, 3 meat, 1 1/2 fat

Sausage, Egg, and Vegetable Casserole

352 CAL, 7 G CARB

1	lb sweet Italian sausage, casing removed, cut into 1" pieces
1	Tbsp + 1½ tsp olive oil
½	sm head escarole, chopped
2	zucchini, thinly sliced
1	red bell pepper, chopped
1	sm red onion, thinly sliced
¼	tsp salt
¼	tsp ground black pepper
7	lg eggs, at room temperature
½	c 2% milk, at room temperature
¼	c grated Parmesan cheese

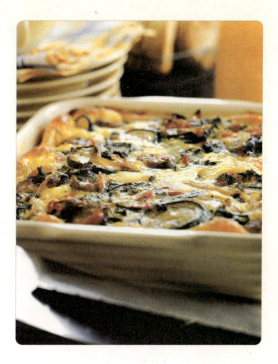

1. Preheat the oven to 350°F. Coat an 8" × 8" baking dish with cooking spray.

2. Cook the sausage in a large skillet over medium-high heat until half-cooked, 6 to 8 minutes, stirring occasionally. Spread over the bottom of the prepared dish. Discard the fat in the skillet. Pour the oil into the same skillet, and stir in the escarole, zucchini, bell pepper, onion, salt, and ⅛ teaspoon of the black pepper. Reduce the heat to medium. Cook, stirring occasionally, until the vegetables are tender and the liquid evaporates, 8 to 10 minutes. Let cool for 10 minutes, and arrange over the sausage.

3. Meanwhile, in a large bowl, combine the eggs, milk, cheese, and the remaining ⅛ teaspoon black pepper. Pour over the vegetables. Bake until the eggs are set, 40 to 45 minutes. Cut into squares to serve. **Makes 6 servings**

PER SERVING: 352 cal, 23 g pro, 7 g carb, 26 g fat, 7 g sat. fat, 308 mg chol, 2 g fiber, 657 mg sodium
DIET EXCHANGES: 0 milk, 1 vegetable, 0 fruit, 0 bread, 3 meat, 3½ fat

Turkey Sandwich with Swiss Cheese and Apple

384 CAL, 28 G CARB

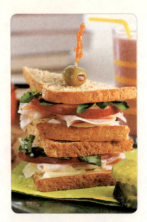

 3 Tbsp macadamia or other nut butter

 8 slices light whole wheat bread, lightly toasted

 4 slices (¼ lb) Swiss cheese

 8 slices (½ lb) cooked turkey breast

¼ tsp salt

⅛ tsp ground black pepper (optional)

 1 sm apple, thinly sliced

½ bunch watercress sprigs or 4 lg lettuce leaves

Spread the nut butter over the bread. Arrange the cheese on 4 slices, top with the turkey, and season with the salt and pepper (if using). Top with the apple, watercress, and the remaining bread. Cut in half. **Makes 4 servings**

PER SERVING: 384 cal, 29 g pro, 28 g carb, 19 g fat, 5 g sat. fat, 60 mg chol, 2 g fiber, 714 mg sodium

DIET EXCHANGES: 0 milk, 0 vegetable, ½ fruit, 2 bread, 3 meat, 1½ fat

Two-Cheese Pita Melt

230 CAL, 19 G CARB

 4 mini whole wheat pitas, split

 4 tsp Dijon mustard

 4 thin slices mozzarella cheese

 4 thin slices Swiss cheese

1⅓ c sliced red or green cabbage

½ tsp dried oregano

½ tsp garlic powder (optional)

¼ tsp salt

¼ tsp ground black pepper

1. Preheat the oven to 400°F.

2. Spread the inside of the pitas with the mustard, and arrange the mozzarella and Swiss cheeses inside.

3. In a bowl, toss the cabbage, oregano, garlic powder (if using), salt, and pepper. Stuff into the pitas. Arrange on a baking sheet, and bake until the cheese melts and the edges of the pitas are crisp, 12 to 15 minutes. **Makes 4 servings**

PER SERVING: 230 cal, 14 g pro, 19 g carb, 12 g fat, 7 g sat. fat, 36 mg chol, 3 g fiber, 562 mg sodium

DIET EXCHANGES: 0 milk, ½ vegetable, 0 fruit, 1 bread, 1½ meat, 1½ fat

Open-Face
Bacon-Mushroom Melt

295 CAL, 14 G CARB

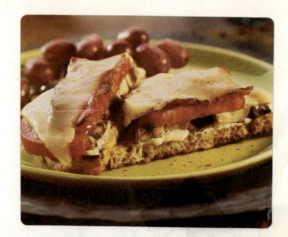

8	strips turkey bacon or pork bacon, halved
4	slices light whole wheat bread, toasted
2	Tbsp mayonnaise
4	mushrooms (4 oz), thinly sliced
⅛	tsp salt
¼	tsp black pepper
4	slices tomato
⅓	lb Muenster cheese, sliced
1	c alfalfa or other sprouts (optional)

1. Place a broiler rack farthest from the heat source, and preheat the broiler (or a toaster oven).

2. Arrange the bacon in a large skillet, and cook over low heat until crisp, turning occasionally, 5 to 8 minutes. Drain on a paper towel–lined plate.

3. Spread the bread with the mayonnaise, and place on a baking sheet. Top with the mushrooms, and season with the salt and pepper. Arrange the tomato over the mushrooms. Cover with slices of the cheese, and top with the bacon.

4. Broil until the cheese melts. Top with the sprouts if using. **Makes 4 servings**

PER SERVING: 295 cal, 16 g pro, 14 g carb, 20 g fat, 9 g sat. fat, 61 mg chol, 1 g fiber, 897 mg sodium

DIET EXCHANGES: 0 milk, 1 vegetable, 0 fruit, ½ bread, 2 meat, 3½ fat

Pesto Chicken Sandwich with Roasted Peppers

328 CAL, 23 G CARB

- 4 whole wheat tortillas (6" diameter)
- ¼ c jarred pesto sauce
- ½ lb sliced chicken breast, warmed
- ¼ tsp salt
- ¼ tsp ground black pepper
- 2 jarred roasted red bell peppers (2 oz), drained and halved
- 4 thin slices (3–4 oz) mozzarella cheese
- 4 romaine lettuce leaves

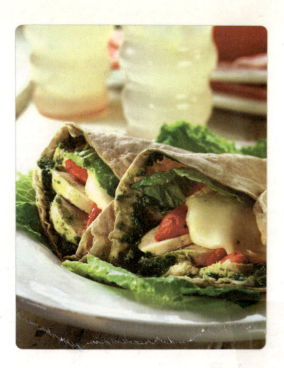

1. Preheat the oven to 350°F.

2. Arrange the tortillas on a baking sheet. Spread the pesto evenly over each. Arrange the chicken in a row down the center of each tortilla, and sprinkle with the salt and black pepper. Top with the roasted peppers and mozzarella.

3. Bake just until heated through and the cheese melts. Top with the lettuce, roll into a cylinder, and serve. **Makes 4 servings**

PER SERVING: 328 cal, 29 g pro, 23 g carb, 16 g fat, 6 g sat. fat, 75 mg chol, 3 g fiber, 598 mg sodium
DIET EXCHANGES: 0 milk, ½ vegetable, 0 fruit, 1½ bread, 3 meat, 2½ fat

Creamy Broccoli Soup with Chicken

177 CAL, 13 G CARB

- 2 Tbsp butter
- 1 onion, thinly sliced
- 1 clove garlic, sliced (optional)
- 3 Tbsp whole wheat flour
- 3 cans (14½ oz each) reduced-sodium chicken broth
- 1½ bunches (1½ lb) broccoli, cut into florets, stems peeled and thinly sliced
- ¾ tsp dried sage
- 1 bay leaf
- ¼ tsp black pepper
- 1 boneless, skinless chicken breast half (½ lb), cut into chunks
- ⅓ c half-and-half

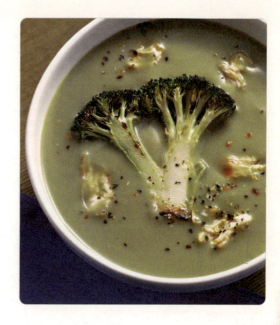

1. Melt the butter in a soup pot over low heat. Stir in the onion and garlic if using. Cover, and cook until the onion is almost translucent, 8 to 10 minutes, stirring occasionally.

2. Stir in the flour, and cook, stirring frequently, for 1 minute. Gradually stir in the broth, bring the soup to a simmer over medium heat, and add the broccoli, sage, and bay leaf. Cook until the broccoli is tender, 10 to 15 minutes.

3. Discard the bay leaf. Reserve ½ cup broccoli florets, if desired. Ladle the soup into a blender, process until smooth, and return to the pot.

4. Add the pepper, chicken, and half-and-half. Cook just until the chicken is no longer pink, 3 to 4 minutes, stirring once or twice. Top each serving with the reserved broccoli florets if using. **Makes 6 servings**

PER SERVING: 177 cal, 16 g pro, 13 g carb, 7 g fat, 4 g sat. fat, 42 mg chol, 4 g fiber, 190 mg sodium

DIET EXCHANGES: 0 milk, 1½ vegetable, 0 fruit, ½ bread, 1 meat, 1 fat

CHAPTER 19

Savory Dinners

One bite of these filling, flavorful dishes, and you'll never look at low-carb the same way again

Spanish-Style Green Beans

162 CAL, 13 G CARB

- 16 oz green beans, trimmed and cut into 2" lengths
- 3 Tbsp olive oil
- 1 onion, chopped
- 1 sm green bell pepper, chopped
- 1 tomato, peeled, seeded, and coarsely chopped
- 2 cloves garlic, minced
- ¼ tsp salt
- ⅛ tsp ground black pepper
- 2–3 Tbsp coarsely chopped, pitted kalamata olives
- 2 tsp drained capers (optional)

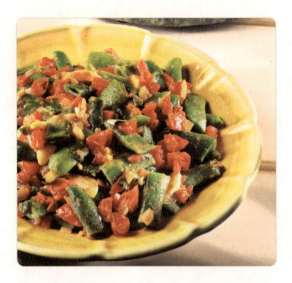

1. Combine the beans, oil, onion, bell pepper, tomato, garlic, salt, and black pepper in a saucepan over medium heat. Cook, stirring, until the vegetables start to sizzle, 2 to 3 minutes.

2. Reduce the heat to low, cover, and cook, stirring occasionally, until the beans are very tender but not falling apart, 20 to 25 minutes. Stir in the olives and capers (if using), and heat for 1 minute. Serve warm, at room temperature, or chilled. **Makes 4 servings**

PER SERVING: 162 cal, 2 g pro, 13 g carb, 12 g fat, 2 g sat. fat, 0 mg chol, 6 g fiber, 230 mg sodium

DIET EXCHANGES: 0 milk, 2½ vegetable, 0 fruit, 0 bread, 0 meat, 2½ fat

Pork Chops Baked with Cabbage and Cream

463 CAL, 12 G CARB

- 1 sm head (1½ lb) green cabbage, cored and finely shredded
- 4 boneless pork chops (6 oz each), ¾" thick
- ½ tsp salt
- ¼ tsp ground black pepper
- 2 tsp olive oil
- ½ c half-and-half
- 1 tsp caraway seeds
- ½ tsp sweet Hungarian paprika
- 1 tsp dried marjoram or thyme
- ½ c (2 oz) shredded Swiss cheese

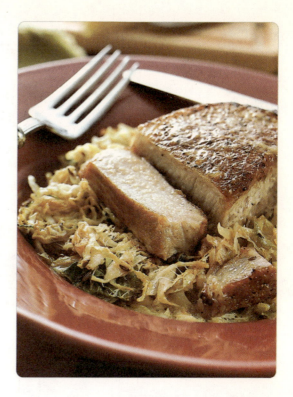

1. Preheat the oven to 350°F.

2. Bring a large pot of salted water to a boil over high heat. Add the cabbage, and cook until soft, 4 to 5 minutes. Drain in a colander, and dry it well with paper towels.

3. Season the meat with ¼ teaspoon of the salt and the pepper. Heat the oil in a large, oven-proof, heavy skillet over high heat. Add the meat, and cook just until browned, 1 to 2 minutes. Remove to a plate.

4. Discard any fat in the skillet, and heat the skillet over low heat. Stir in the cabbage, half-and-half, caraway seeds, paprika, marjoram, and the remaining ¼ teaspoon salt. Cook, stirring, until heated through, about 1 minute. Remove from the heat, and arrange the pork over the cabbage, adding any accumulated juices. Sprinkle with the cheese. Bake until a meat thermometer registers 160°F for medium-well, about 25 minutes.

Makes 4 servings

PER SERVING: 463 cal, 53 g pro, 12 g carb, 20 g fat, 9 g sat. fat, 165 mg chol, 4 g fiber, 460 mg sodium

DIET EXCHANGES: 0 milk, 2½ vegetable, 0 fruit, 0 bread, 7 meat, 3½ fat

Stir-Fried Chicken and Broccoli

321 CAL, 18 G CARB

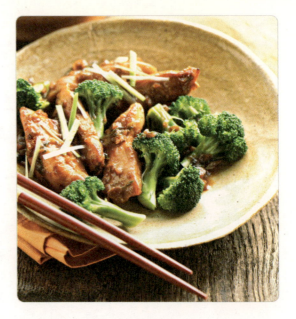

1/2 c chicken broth

3 Tbsp Chinese oyster sauce

2 Tbsp orange juice

1 Tbsp + 1 1/2 tsp soy sauce

2 cloves garlic, minced

2 tsp minced fresh ginger

1 tsp sesame oil

1/4 tsp hot-pepper sauce (optional)

1 Tbsp cornstarch

1 Tbsp + 1 1/2 tsp cold water

3 Tbsp vegetable oil

1 lb boneless, skinless chicken breasts, cut into thin strips

1 lg bunch (2 lb) broccoli, cut into sm florets

5 scallions, minced

1 tsp toasted sesame seeds (optional)

1. In a small bowl, combine the broth, oyster sauce, orange juice, soy sauce, garlic, ginger, sesame oil, and hot-pepper sauce (if using).

2. In a cup, dissolve the cornstarch in the water.

3. Heat the vegetable oil in a large wok or skillet over high heat until the oil just starts to smoke. Add the chicken, and cook, stirring continually, until no longer pink on the surface, about 30 seconds. Stir in the broccoli, and cook, stirring continually, until it turns bright green and the chicken is half cooked, about 2 minutes. Pour in the broth mixture, and cook, stirring frequently, for 2 minutes. Stir in the scallions and cornstarch mixture. Cook, stirring, until the sauce comes to a boil, thickens, and the chicken is cooked through, about 1 minute.

4. Sprinkle with the sesame seeds (if using).

Makes 4 servings

PER SERVING: *321 cal, 34 g pro, 18 g carb, 14 g fat, 1 g sat. fat, 66 mg chol, 8 g fiber, 692 mg sodium*

DIET EXCHANGES: 0 milk, 3 vegetable, 0 fruit, 0 bread, 4 meat, 2 1/2 fat

Breaded Baked Cod with Tartar Sauce

268 CAL, 14 G CARB

Tarter Sauce

- ¹/₂ c reduced-fat mayonnaise
- 1¹/₂ Tbsp lemon juice
- 1 Tbsp finely chopped dill or sweet pickle
- 2 tsp mustard
- 2 tsp capers, drained and chopped
- 2 tsp chopped parsley (optional)

Fish

- 2 slices whole wheat bread, torn
- 2 eggs
- 1 Tbsp water
- 1¹/₄ lb cod or scrod fillet, cut into 1"–1¹/₂" pieces
- ¹/₂ tsp salt
- ¹/₄ tsp ground black pepper

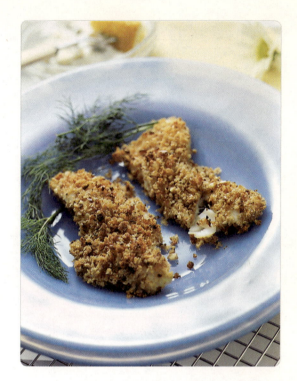

1. *To make the tartar sauce:* In a small bowl, combine the mayonnaise, lemon juice, pickle, mustard, capers, and parsley (if using). Cover, and refrigerate.

2. *To make the fish:* Preheat the oven to 400°F. Coat a baking sheet with cooking spray.

3. Place the bread in a food processor, and process into fine crumbs. Place in a shallow bowl. In another bowl, beat the eggs with the water. Season the fish with the salt and pepper. Dip the fish into the eggs, then into the breadcrumbs. Place on the prepared baking sheet. Generously coat the breaded fish with cooking spray. Bake until opaque inside, about 10 minutes. Serve with the tartar sauce. **Makes 4 servings**

PER SERVING: 268 cal, 30 g pro, 14 g carb, 10 g fat, 2 g sat. fat, 174 mg chol, 1 g fiber, 734 mg sodium

DIET EXCHANGES: 0 milk, 0 vegetable, 0 fruit, 1 bread, 3¹/₂ meat, ¹/₂ fat

Mushroom and Kasha Soup

112 CAL, 11 G CARB

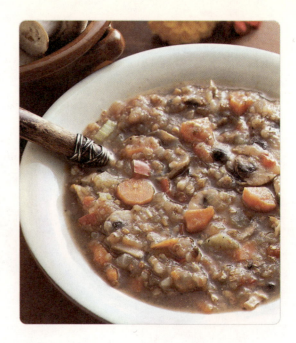

½ c kasha (buckwheat groats)

2 Tbsp olive oil

20 oz mushrooms, coarsely chopped

½ onion, finely chopped

1 carrot, finely chopped

1½ ribs celery, finely chopped

½ red bell pepper, finely chopped

½ tsp ground black pepper

2¼ cans (14½ oz each) chicken or vegetable broth

1 tsp dried dill or thyme

1 bay leaf

1. Toast the kasha in a soup pot over medium heat, stirring, for 2 to 3 minutes. Remove to a bowl.

2. Heat the oil in the same pot over medium-low heat. Stir in the mushrooms, onion, carrot, celery, bell pepper, and black pepper. Cover, and cook, stirring occasionally, for 8 to 10 minutes.

3. Stir in the kasha and broth. Bring to a simmer, and add the dill and bay leaf. Partially cover, and cook until the kasha is tender, about 10 minutes. Remove the bay leaf before serving.
Makes 6 servings

PER SERVING: 112 cal, 6 g pro, 11 g carb, 6 g fat, 1 g sat. fat, 0 mg chol, 3 g fiber, 687 mg sodium

DIET EXCHANGES: 0 milk, 1½ vegetable, 0 fruit, ½ bread, 0 meat, 1 fat

Scallops in Tarragon Cream

201 CAL, 5 G CARB

  1 Tbsp butter, softened

1½ lb fresh or thawed frozen sea scallops, rinsed

1½ tsp chopped fresh tarragon or ½ tsp dried

  ¼ tsp ground black pepper

  ¼ c half-and-half

  1 Tbsp Pernod or 2 Tbsp dry sherry (optional)

  2 Tbsp lemon juice

  1 Tbsp chopped parsley

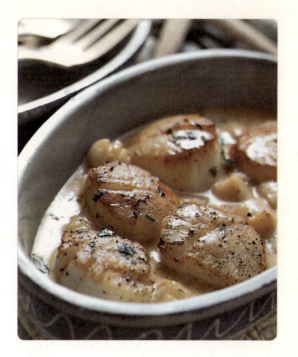

1. Melt the butter in a large skillet over medium-high heat. When the butter foams, add the scallops, tarragon, and pepper. Cook for 2 to 3 minutes, stirring constantly.

   2. Stir in the half-and-half, Pernod (if using), and lemon juice. Reduce the heat to medium-low, and cook until the scallops look opaque throughout and feel slightly springy when lightly pressed, 1 to 2 minutes.

   3. Stir in the parsley. **Makes 4 servings**

PER SERVING: 201 cal, 29 g pro, 5 g carb, 6 g fat, 3 g sat. fat, 71 mg chol, 0 g fiber, 312 mg sodium

DIET EXCHANGES: 0 milk, 0 vegetable, 0 fruit, 0 bread, 4 meat, 1 fat

Filet Mignon with Tomatoes and Rosemary

303 CAL, 3 G CARB

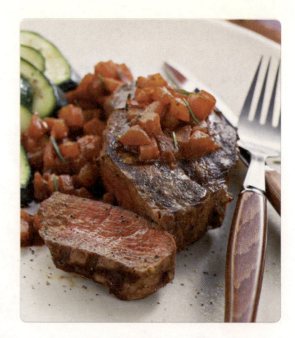

2	tsp soy sauce
1½	tsp Dijon mustard
1½	tsp chopped fresh rosemary or ½ tsp dried and crumbled
⅛	tsp garlic powder
2	tomatoes, finely chopped
2	tsp olive oil
4	filet mignons (6 oz each), 1½" thick
¼	tsp salt
½	tsp ground black pepper

1. Preheat the oven to 400°F.

2. In a bowl, combine the soy sauce, mustard, rosemary, and garlic powder. Fold in the tomatoes.

3. Heat the oil in a large, oven-safe, heavy skillet over high heat. Season the meat with the salt and pepper. Place it in the skillet, and deeply brown the first side, 4 to 5 minutes. Turn, and brown the second side for 30 seconds. Place the skillet in the oven, and cook until a meat thermometer registers 145°F for medium rare, 12 to 14 minutes. Serve topped with the tomatoes. **Makes 4 servings**

PER SERVING: 303 cal, 37 g pro, 3 g carb, 15 g fat, 5 g sat. fat, 105 mg chol, 1 g fiber, 430 mg sodium

DIET EXCHANGES: 0 milk, ½ vegetable, 0 fruit, 0 bread, 5 meat, ½ fat

Smothered Pot Roast

417 CAL, 8 G CARB

 1 Tbsp + 1¹/₂ tsp olive oil
 1 med onion, cut into sm wedges
 2 cloves garlic, minced
 1 boneless beef chuck (about 2 lb)
¹/₄ tsp salt
¹/₂ tsp black pepper
1¹/₂ tsp whole wheat flour
 1 can (14¹/₂ oz) beef broth
 1 can (6 oz) vegetable cocktail juice
 1 tsp Worcestershire sauce
¹/₂ tsp dried thyme

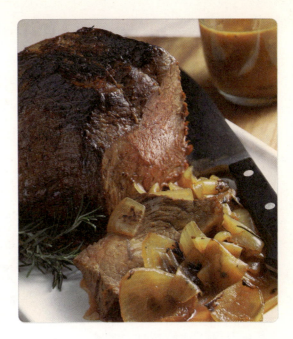

1. Preheat the oven to 350°F.

2. Heat 1 tablespoon of the oil in a large, heavy pot with ovenproof handles over medium heat. Add the onion and garlic. Cover, and cook, stirring occasionally, until the onion begins to brown and turn translucent, 5 to 8 minutes. Remove to a plate. Remove the pot from the heat.

3. Season the meat with the salt and pepper, and sprinkle all over with the flour, rubbing it in lightly. Heat the remaining 1¹/₂ teaspoons oil in the pot over high heat. Add the meat, and cook until browned, 3 to 5 minutes.

4. Reduce the heat to low, and return the vegetables to the pot, scattering them over and around the meat. Add the broth, juice, Worcestershire, and thyme. Bring to a simmer, and cover. Bake until fork-tender, 2 to 2¹/₂ hours.

5. Remove the beef and vegetables to a platter. Pour the pan juices into a fat separator or glass cup, and discard the fat that rises to the surface. Pour the juices over the meat, and serve. **Makes 4 servings**

PER SERVING: 417 cal, 53 g pro, 8 g carb, 18 g fat, 6 g sat. fat, 155 mg chol, 1 g fiber, 738 mg sodium

DIET EXCHANGES: 0 milk, 1 vegetable, 0 fruit, 0 bread, 6¹/₂ meat, 1 fat

Meat Loaf with Walnuts

222 CAL, 7 G CARB

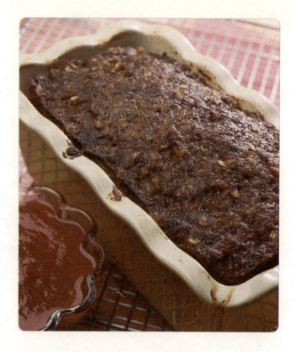

- 1 lg egg, lightly beaten
- 2 Tbsp Worcestershire sauce
- ¹/₄ c tomato paste
- ¹/₂ tsp dried thyme
- ¹/₂ tsp salt
- ¹/₂ tsp black pepper
- ¹/₂ med onion, finely chopped
- 1 lg clove garlic, minced
- ²/₃ c (1¹/₂ oz) ground walnuts
- 1¹/₂ lb extralean ground beef chuck
- ¹/₂ c tomato sauce

1. Preheat the oven to 375°F.

2. In a large bowl, combine the egg, Worcestershire, tomato paste, thyme, salt, and pepper. Add the onion, garlic, walnuts, and beef. Using a fork, gently combine the meat with the seasonings.

3. Form into a loaf, and place in a 9" × 5" × 3" loaf pan. Spread the tomato sauce evenly over the top. Bake until the juices run clear and a meat thermometer registers 160°F, 50 to 55 minutes. Pour off the fat in the pan, and slice the loaf. **Makes 6 servings**

PER SERVING: 222 cal, 26 g pro, 7 g carb, 11 g fat, 3 g sat. fat, 95 mg chol, 1 g fiber, 430 mg sodium

DIET EXCHANGES: 0 milk, 1 vegetable, 0 fruit, 0 bread, 4 meat, 1½ fat

Chicken Parmesan

366 CAL, 16 G CARB

Sauce

1 Tbsp olive oil

2 cloves garlic, minced

1¼ c canned crushed tomatoes

2 Tbsp Italian-style tomato paste

⅛ tsp dried oregano

⅛ tsp dried basil

¼ tsp salt

⅛ tsp black pepper

Chicken

6 slices light whole wheat bread

2 lg eggs

2 Tbsp water

4 boneless, skinless chicken breast halves (6 oz each), pounded to ¼" thickness

¼ tsp salt

½ tsp black pepper

¼ c soy flour or whole wheat flour

2 tsp olive oil

6 oz shredded part-skim mozzarella cheese

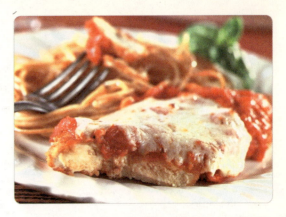

1. *To make the sauce:* Heat the oil in a small saucepan over low heat. Stir in the garlic, and cook, stirring frequently, for 30 seconds. Add the tomatoes, tomato paste, oregano, and basil. Cook until thick and rich, 12 to 15 minutes, stirring occasionally. Season with the salt and pepper. Cover, and keep warm.

2. *To make the chicken:* While the sauce is cooking, preheat the oven to 250°F. Place the bread on a baking sheet, and bake until completely dry, 10 to 12 minutes. Let cool slightly. Transfer the bread to a food processor, and grind to make about 1 cup of crumbs. Remove to a large plate.

3. In a shallow bowl, lightly beat the eggs with the water. Season the chicken with the salt and pepper, and coat with the flour. Dip into the egg mixture, then press into the crumbs to coat both sides.

4. Place the broiler rack 4" to 5" from the heat, and preheat the broiler.

5. Heat 1 teaspoon of the oil in a large skillet over medium heat. Add 2 of the coated chicken breasts, and cook until golden brown on one side, 2 to 3 minutes. Turn, and cook until no longer pink and the juices run clear, 2 to 3 minutes. Remove to a 13" × 9" baking dish. Repeat with the remaining 1 teaspoon oil and remaining chicken.

6. Top with the sauce, and sprinkle with the cheese. Broil just until the cheese melts, 1 to 2 minutes. **Makes 6 servings**

PER SERVING: 366 cal, 40 g pro, 16 g carb, 16 g fat, 5 g sat. fat, 153 mg chol, 2 g fiber, 572 mg sodium

DIET EXCHANGES: 0 milk, ½ vegetable, 0 fruit, 1 bread, 5 meat, 2 fat

Turkey Cutlets with Ham and Provolone

362 CAL, 4 G CARB

- 4 turkey cutlets (4 oz each)
- ½ tsp salt
- ¼ tsp black pepper
- ¼ c soy flour
- 1 Tbsp olive oil
- 4 thin slices (3 oz total) ham, cut in half
- 4 thin slices (4 oz total) provolone cheese, cut in half
- 4 lemon wedges

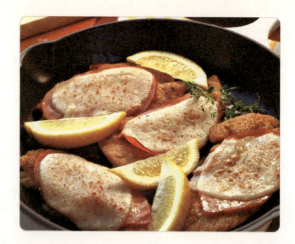

1. Season the turkey with the salt and pepper. Coat in the flour, and pat off the excess.

2. Heat the oil in a large nonstick skillet over high heat. Add the turkey, and cook until browned on one side, 2 to 3 minutes. Turn, reduce the heat to low, and layer the ham and cheese on top. Cover, and cook until the turkey juices run clear and the cheese melts, 2 to 3 minutes. Serve immediately with the lemon wedges for squeezing. **Makes 4 servings**

PER SERVING: 362 cal, 39 g pro, 4 g carb, 20 g fat, 8 g sat. fat, 105 mg chol, 1 g fiber, 479 mg sodium

DIET EXCHANGES: 0 milk, 0 vegetable, 0 fruit, ½ bread, 5½ meat, 2½ fat

CHAPTER 20

Just Desserts

These yummy treats prove that low-carb dieters can have their cake (and pudding and cookies) and their waistline too

Cantaloupe Sorbet

61 CAL, 15 G CARB

4	c frozen cantaloupe, slightly thawed
1	frozen banana, sliced
¼	c Splenda
1	Tbsp crème de menthe liqueur (optional)
1	Tbsp lime juice
2	tsp grated lime peel
⅛–¼	tsp ground cinnamon

1. In a food processor, combine the cantaloupe, banana, Splenda, liqueur (if using), lime juice, lime peel, and cinnamon. Process until smooth.

2. Scrape into a shallow metal pan. Cover, and freeze for 4 hours or overnight. Using a knife, break the mixture into chunks. Process briefly in a food processor before serving. **Makes 6 servings**

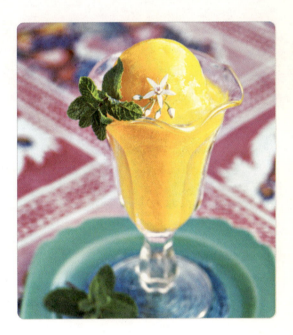

PER SERVING: 61 cal, 1 g pro, 15 g carb, 0 g fat, 0 g sat. fat, 0 mg cholesterol, 2 g fiber, 11 mg sodium

DIET EXCHANGES: 0 milk, 0 vegetable, 1 fruit, 0 bread, 0 meat, 0 fat

Orange-Walnut Biscotti

76 CAL, 8 G CARB

^{2}/$_3$ c walnuts

^{1}/$_4$ c sugar

1^1/$_4$ c whole grain pastry flour

^{1}/$_4$ c cornmeal

1 tsp baking powder

^{1}/$_4$ tsp salt

^{1}/$_4$ c butter, softened

^{1}/$_4$ c Splenda

2 eggs

2 tsp grated orange peel

^{1}/$_2$ tsp orange extract

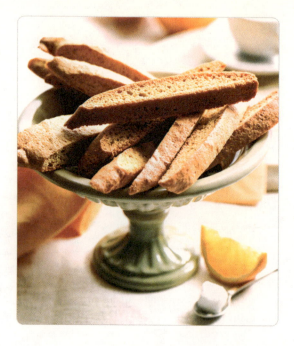

1. In a food processor, combine the walnuts and 2 tablespoons of the sugar. Process until the walnuts are coarsely ground but not made into a paste. Transfer to a large bowl, and add the flour, cornmeal, baking powder, and salt. Stir until combined.

2. In a large bowl, using an electric mixer, beat the butter, Splenda, and the remaining 2 tablespoons sugar until light and fluffy. Beat in the eggs, orange peel, and orange extract. Gradually beat in the flour mixture until smooth and thick. Divide the dough into two equal-size pieces. Refrigerate for 30 minutes, or until firm.

3. Preheat the oven to 350°F. Coat a baking sheet with cooking spray.

4. Shape each piece of dough into a 12"-long log, and place both on the prepared baking sheet. Bake for 25 to 30 minutes, or until golden. Remove the logs to racks to cool.

5. Cut each log on a slight diagonal into ^{1}/$_2$"-thick slices. Place the slices, cut side down, on the baking sheet, and bake for 5 minutes. Turn the slices over, and bake for 5 minutes longer, or until dry. Remove to racks to cool. **Makes 24**

PER BISCOTTO: 76 cal, 2 g pro, 8 g carb, 5 g fat, 2 g sat. fat, 23 mg cholesterol, 1 g fiber, 68 mg sodium

DIET EXCHANGES: 0 milk, 0 vegetable, 0 fruit, ^{1}/$_2$ bread, 0 meat, 1 fat

Peanut Butter Cookies

94 CAL, 7 G CARB

- 6 Tbsp unsalted butter, softened
- $^1/_2$ c unsweetened smooth peanut butter, at room temperature
- $^1/_4$ c packed light brown sugar
- $^1/_4$ c Splenda
- 1 lg egg, at room temperature, lightly beaten
- 1 tsp vanilla extract
- 1$^1/_4$ c sifted oat flour
- $^1/_4$ tsp baking powder
- 3 Tbsp salted peanuts, chopped

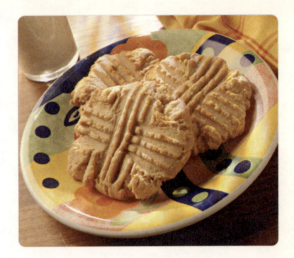

1. Place an oven rack in the middle position, and preheat the oven to 350°F.

2. In a large bowl, beat together the butter and peanut butter until very smooth, about 1 minute. Add the brown sugar and Splenda, and beat until well combined and light in color, 1 to 2 minutes. Gradually beat in the egg and vanilla extract, beating until very smooth and a little fluffy, 1 to 2 minutes. Mix in the flour and baking powder, beating until a moist but cohesive dough forms. Stir in the peanuts.

3. Drop by the tablespoon about 2" apart on nonstick baking sheets. Using the tines of a fork dampened in cold water, flatten each in a cross-hatch pattern until 2" in diameter. Bake until golden brown, 22 to 25 minutes. Remove to a rack to cool. **Makes 24**

PER COOKIE: 94 cal, 3 g pro, 7 g carb, 7 g fat, 2 g sat. fat, 17 mg chol, 1 g fiber, 56 mg sodium

DIET EXCHANGES: 0 milk, 0 vegetable, 0 fruit, ½ bread, ½ meat, 1 fat

Gingerbread Cake with Peach Whipped Cream

238 CAL, 25 G CARB

1½ c sifted oat flour

¾ c whole grain pastry flour

2 tsp baking powder

1 tsp ground ginger

1 tsp ground cinnamon

½ tsp ground cloves

Pinch of salt

¼ c light molasses

⅓ c vegetable oil

1¼ c hot water

1 tsp baking soda

1 lg egg + 1 yolk, at room temperature, lightly beaten

¼ tsp liquid stevia or ¼ c Splenda

½ c heavy cream

3 Tbsp peach fruit spread, at room temperature

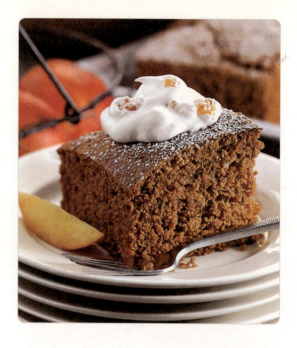

1. Preheat the oven to 350°F. Coat an 8" round cake pan with cooking spray.

2. In a medium bowl, combine the flours, baking powder, ginger, cinnamon, cloves, and salt.

3. In a large bowl, combine the molasses and oil. In a 2-cup glass measure, combine the water and baking soda. Whisk into the molasses mixture.

4. Gradually whisk the dry ingredients into the molasses mixture. Whisk in the egg, yolk, and stevia. Pour into the prepared pan, and bake until a toothpick inserted in the center comes out clean, about 30 minutes.

5. Cool in the pan on a rack for 10 minutes. Remove to the rack, and let cool completely.

6. In a large bowl, whip the cream and fruit spread together until firm but soft peaks form. Serve wedges of cake topped with a spoonful of the peach cream. **Makes 10 servings**

PER SERVING: 238 cal, 4 g pro, 25 g carb, 14 g fat, 4 g sat. fat, 59 mg chol, 3 g fiber, 262 mg sodium

DIET EXCHANGES: 0 milk, 0 vegetable, 0 fruit, 1½ bread, 0 meat, 2½ fat

Strawberry Cream Cake

273 CAL, 24 G CARB

Cake

- ³/₄ c sifted whole wheat pastry flour
- ³/₄ c sifted oat flour
- 1 Tbsp baking powder
- ¹/₂ c butter, slightly softened
- ¹/₄ c packed brown sugar
- ¹/₄ c Splenda
- 2 egg yolks + 3 whites, at room temperature
- ³/₄ c 2% milk, at room temperature
- 1 tsp vanilla extract

Topping

- ³/₄ c heavy cream
- ¹/₄ c strawberry all-fruit spread
- 1 pt strawberries, hulled and sliced

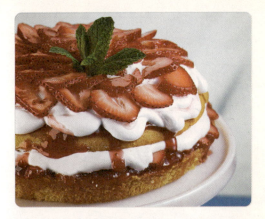

1. *To make the cake:* Preheat the oven to 350°F. Butter and flour an 8" round cake pan or an 8" × 8" baking pan.

2. In a small bowl, combine the pastry flour, oat flour, and baking powder.

3. In a large bowl, using an electric mixer on medium speed, beat the butter, sugar, and Splenda until creamy, about 2 minutes. Add the egg yolks, one at a time, beating until the mixture is somewhat fluffy, 3 to 4 minutes.

4. Beat in the flour mixture alternately with the milk in 3 additions. Beat in the vanilla extract.

5. In a clean, large bowl, beat the 3 egg whites until they form stiff but moist peaks, about 1 minute. Spoon one-third of the whites on top of the egg yolk mixture, and gently fold in. Fold in the remaining whites. Spoon into the prepared pan, and bake until a toothpick inserted in the center comes out clean, 35 to 40 minutes.

6. Cool in the pan on a rack for 10 to 15 minutes. Remove to the rack, and cool completely.

7. *To make the topping:* In a clean, large bowl, whip the cream until firm but soft peaks form, and refrigerate.

8. Melt the all-fruit spread in a small skillet over very low heat, stirring, about 15 seconds. To make a layer cake, split the completely cooled cake horizontally into 2 layers. Spread one-third of the fruit spread over the cut side of the bottom layer. Cover with one-third of the whipped cream and one-third of the berries. Top with the remaining layer, and coat with the remaining fruit spread and whipped cream. Arrange the remaining berries over the top. **Makes 10 servings**

PER SERVING: 273 cal, 5 g pro, 24 g carb, 18 g fat, 10 g sat. fat, 93 mg cholesterol, 2 g fiber, 253 mg sodium

DIET EXCHANGES: 0 milk, 0 vegetable, ½ fruit, 1 bread, ½ meat, 3½ fat

Double Chocolate Pudding

142 CAL, 23 G CARB

- 1/3 c packed brown sugar
- 1/3 c Splenda
- 1/4 c unsweetened cocoa powder
- 2 Tbsp cornstarch
- 2 c whole milk or unsweetened soy milk
- 1 oz bittersweet chocolate
- 1 tsp vanilla extract

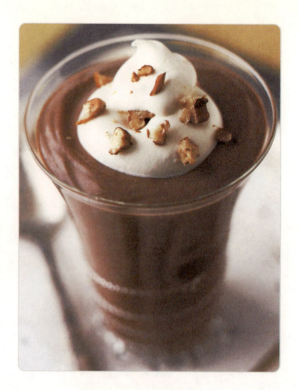

1. In a medium saucepan, whisk together the brown sugar, Splenda, cocoa, and cornstarch until smooth. Whisk in the milk over medium heat. Cook until thickened and bubbly, about 2 minutes. Remove from the heat, and stir in the chocolate and vanilla extract. Stir until the chocolate melts.

2. Pour into 4 custard cups or small serving dishes. Cover with plastic wrap, and chill for 2 hours before serving. **Makes 6 servings**

PER SERVING: 142 cal, 4 g pro, 23 g carb, 5 g fat, 3 g sat. fat, 11 mg chol, 2 g fiber, 46 mg sodium

DIET EXCHANGES: 1/2 milk, 0 vegetable, 0 fruit, 1 bread, 0 meat, 1/2 fat

FIT TIP! Keep treats on hand

If you have a sweet tooth, make the cookies and desserts in this book that keep well so that they are ready when you need them. Keep sugar-free gelatin in the refrigerator, and top with a couple of squirts of canned real whipped cream. Or look in your local supermarket or health food store for low-carbohydrate chocolate snack bars, cookies, cake mixes, milkshakes, and beverages.

Raspberry-Almond Tart

138 CAL, 21 G CARB

Crust

- 2/3 c old-fashioned or quick-cooking rolled oats
- 1/2 c whole grain pastry flour
- 1 Tbsp sugar
- 1 tsp ground cinnamon
- 1/4 tsp baking soda
- 2 Tbsp canola oil
- 2–3 Tbsp plain yogurt
- 1/3 c semisweet mini–chocolate chips (optional)

Filling

- 1/4 c raspberry all-fruit spread
- 3/4 tsp almond extract
- 2 1/2 c raspberries
- 2 Tbsp sliced almonds

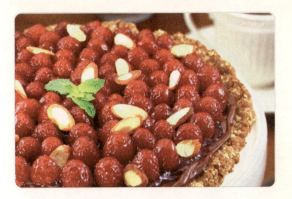

1. *To make the crust:* Preheat the oven to 375°F. Coat a baking sheet with cooking spray.

2. In a medium bowl, combine the oats, flour, sugar, cinnamon, and baking soda. Stir in the oil and 2 tablespoons of the yogurt to make a soft, slightly sticky dough. If the dough is too stiff, add the remaining 1 tablespoon yogurt.

3. Place the dough on the prepared baking sheet and, using lightly oiled hands, pat evenly into a 10" circle.

4. Place a 9" cake pan right side up on the dough, and trace around the bottom of the pan with a sharp knife, being careful only to score the surface of the dough. With your fingers, push up and pinch the dough around the outside of the pan to make a 9" crust with a rim 1/4" high. Remove the cake pan. Bake for 12 minutes on the baking sheet. Scatter the chocolate chips (if using) evenly over the surface of the crust, and bake until the chocolate is melted and the crust is firm and golden, 3 to 4 minutes longer. Remove from the oven, and spread the chocolate over the crust to make an even layer. Set aside to cool.

5. *To make the filling:* In a small, microwaveable bowl, combine the all-fruit spread and almond extract. Microwave on high for 10 to 15 seconds, or until melted. Brush a generous tablespoon evenly over the crust. Arrange the raspberries evenly over the crust. Brush the remaining spread evenly over the berries, making sure to get some of the spread between the berries to secure them. Sprinkle with the almonds. Refrigerate for at least 30 minutes, or until the spread has jelled.

Makes 8 servings

PER SERVING: 138 cal, 3 g pro, 21 g carb, 5 g fat, 0 g sat. fat, 0 mg chol, 4 g fiber, 43 mg sodium

DIET EXCHANGES: 0 milk, 0 vegetable, 1/2 fruit, 1/2 bread, 0 meat, 1 fat

Chocolate Hazelnut Flourless Cake

160 CAL, 15 G CARB

 2 Tbsp unsalted butter
 3 Tbsp unsweetened cocoa powder
 ½ c blanched hazelnuts or almonds
 8 Tbsp sugar
 3 oz bittersweet chocolate
 ½ c reduced-fat sour cream
 2 egg yolks
 1 Tbsp Frangelico or amaretto (optional)
 1 tsp vanilla extract
 ½ tsp ground cinnamon
 5 egg whites, at room temperature
 ¼ tsp salt
   Fresh sliced strawberries for serving (optional)

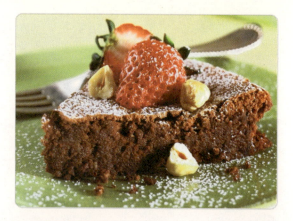

1. Preheat the oven to 350°F. Generously coat an 8" or 9" springform pan with 2 teaspoons of the butter, and dust with 1 tablespoon of the cocoa (don't tap out the excess cocoa; leave it in the pan).

2. In a food processor, combine the nuts with 1 tablespoon of the sugar until finely ground.

3. In the top of a double boiler over barely simmering water, melt the chocolate and the remaining 4 teaspoons butter, stirring occasionally, until smooth.

4. Remove from the heat. Place the chocolate mixture in a large bowl. Add the nut mixture, sour cream, egg yolks, Frangelico (if using), vanilla extract, cinnamon, 5 tablespoons of the remaining sugar, and the remaining 2 tablespoons cocoa. Stir until well blended.

5. In another large bowl, with an electric mixer on high speed, beat the egg whites and salt until foamy. Gradually add the remaining 2 tablespoons sugar, beating, until the whites hold stiff peaks when the beaters are lifted.

6. Stir one-quarter of the beaten whites into the chocolate mixture to lighten it. Gently fold in the remaining whites. Spoon into the prepared pan. Gently smooth the top.

7. Bake for 30 minutes, or until the cake has risen, is dry on the top, and a toothpick inserted in the center comes out with a few moist crumbs. Cool on a rack until warm. The cake will fall dramatically. Loosen the edge of the cake with a knife, and remove the pan side. Serve with the strawberries if using. **Makes 12 servings**

PER SERVING: 160 cal, 4 g pro, 15 g carb, 10 g fat, 4 g sat. fat, 46 mg chol, 1 g fiber, 80 mg sodium
DIET EXCHANGES: 0 milk, 0 vegetable, 0 fruit, 1 bread, 0 meat, 2 fat

Peach Soufflé with Blueberries

96 CAL, 17 G CARB

1$^1/_2$ c frozen peaches, thawed and
         patted dry

   2 Tbsp sugar

   2 Tbsp Splenda

   2 egg yolks

   1 Tbsp lemon juice

$^1/_2$ tsp ground nutmeg

   5 egg whites, at room temperature

$^1/_2$ tsp cream of tartar

$^1/_8$ tsp ground cinnamon

$^1/_2$ c blueberries

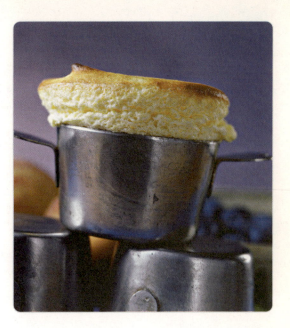

1. Preheat the oven to 350°F.

2. In a blender or food processor, puree the peaches. Transfer to a medium bowl, and stir in the sugar, Splenda, egg yolks, lemon juice, and nutmeg. Set aside.

3. In a large, clean bowl, using an electric mixer, beat the egg whites at medium speed until foamy. Add the cream of tartar, and beat on high speed until stiff peaks form.

4. Stir one-quarter of the egg-white mixture into the peach mixture to lighten it. Gently fold the peach mixture back into the remaining egg-white mixture.

5. Scrape into a 1$^1/_2$-quart soufflé or baking dish, and sprinkle with the cinnamon. Place the dish in a larger dish or baking pan, then place on the bottom rack of the oven. Pour 1" of hot water into the large baking dish or pan. Bake for 50 to 60 minutes, or until puffed and lightly browned. Do not open the oven door during baking. Serve immediately with the blueberries. The soufflé will fall as it cools. **Makes 4 servings**

PER SERVING: 96 cal, 2 g pro, 17 g carb, 12 g fat, 3 g sat. fat, 106 mg chol, 2 g fiber, 5 mg sodium

DIET EXCHANGES: 0 milk, 0 vegetable, 1 fruit, 0 bread, 0 meat, $^1/_2$ fat

All recipes excerpted from the book *Lose Weight the Smart Low-Carb Way* by Bettina Newman, RD, and David Joachim, © 2002 Rodale Inc. Order by calling (800) 848-4735 or visiting www.rodalestore.com.

keep the drive alive!

156 **17 Tips for Putting You First**
Here's how to work out without stressing yourself
(and your family and your boss) out

162 **10 Gotta-Have Workout Toys**
New exercise gadgets can be fun, motivational,
and may even help keep you safe

165 **Workouts to Match Your Mood**
Don't let your emotional ups
and downs sabotage your fitness

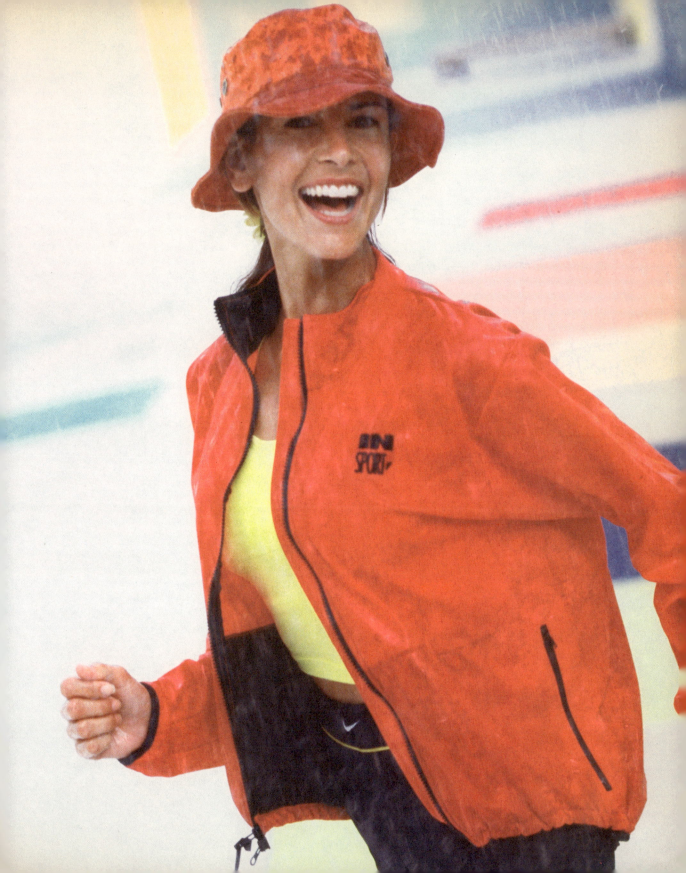

17 Tips for Putting You First

Here's how to work out without stressing yourself (and your family and your boss) out

Maybe it's because everyone acts so darn helpless around us, but women are afraid everything will come crumbling down if they leave their jobs or family for an hour or two of playtime. What they forget is the golden rule of caretaking: You'll be much better equipped to help others if you take care of yourself first. Here are 16 more reasons for making *your* fitness priority number one.

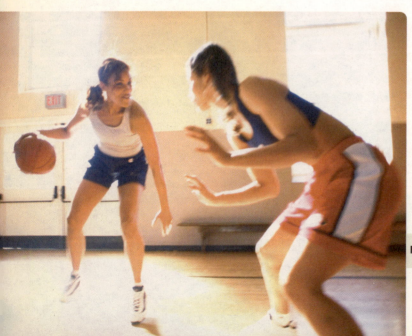

Play more; live happier.

You'll be happier. Regular exercise helps make you happy. Literally hundreds of studies have found that to be true. Researchers at Harvard University found that 10 weeks of strength training actually reduced clinical depression symptoms more successfully than did standard counseling. Psychologists are increasingly prescribing exercise to treat mild to moderate depression as well as anxiety disorders and alcohol abuse. So the next time you're feeling guilty or facing frowns from the family on your way out the door, explain that exercising for 1 hour lifts your mood and makes you more fun to be around when you return.

You'll feel sexier. Women who feel good about their bodies have steamier love lives than those who don't. And women who exercise regularly tend to be happier with their naked selves. What's even better is that vigorous exercise produces feel-good hormones called endorphins that make some women feel sexier after they work out.

He **takes plenty of playtime.** A typical golf game lasts 3 to 4 hours. And the typical guy doesn't wrack himself with guilt about going out to the greens for the afternoon. The same goes for softball, hoops, racquetball, or any other sports that men play. Embrace your active hobbies the same way he embraces his—with guilt-free enthusiasm. To reduce precious weekend time spent apart, try to coordinate your activities so that you're wrapping up at about the same time.

It's problem-solving time. For many women, exercise time is thinking time. In fact, it's the *only* time many working moms get to be alone with their own thoughts. Let your loved ones know that you need this time to think—undisturbed.

You can help a good cause. It's not that you aren't enough of a good cause, but some women feel less guilty about time spent running, walking,

You can get a quality pair of running shoes for the price of one session with a shrink.

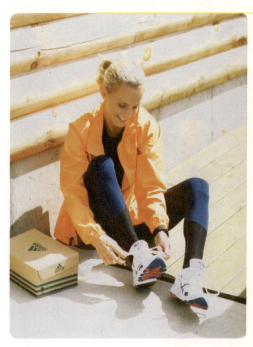

or cycling when they're also benefiting a favorite charity. Signing up for a run, walk, or ride to raise money for multiple sclerosis, diabetes, cancer, or AIDS makes you feel like you're benefiting others as well as yourself.

It's like recess. Your kids don't feel guilty when they want to go out and play; they get excited about it. Let them know that parents like playtime just as much as kids do. They won't always be happy about it, but it's a valuable lesson.

Exercise is cheaper than therapy. Stress raises blood pressure, tightens muscles, interrupts

Cop a New Attitude
Success starts in your head

The best intentions can be undermined by bad attitudes. Here's how to adjust some common thoughts for maximum fitness and weight loss results.

"I WAS BORN TO BE FAT." A USDA study found that women who think their gene pool preordains their jean size were more likely to be heavy. "Genes do have an impact on weight," says Thomas Wadden, PhD, director of the Weight and Eating Disorders Program at the University of Pennsylvania. "But your environment ultimately determines how fat you become." *Attitude adjustment:* "The food and lifestyle choices I make shape my shape."

"I WON'T BE HAPPY *OR* HEALTHY UNTIL I LOSE LOTS OF WEIGHT." Your goal may be too ambitious. "I see patients who want to lose 35% of their initial weight," says Dr. Wadden. "Then they're surprised at how good a 10% loss feels." *Attitude adjustment:* "I'll be happier and healthier if I lose just 10 to 15 lb."

"I DON'T EAT OUT MUCH." Maybe not in the special occasion sense, but every cafeteria lunch, take-out dinner, and vending machine snack still counts as food you don't cook at home. For many of us, dining out is tantamount to pigging out, warns Joanne Guthrie, PhD, RD, a USDA nutritionist. *Attitude adjustment:* "How many calories are hiding in this meal that I didn't make?"

digestion, weakens your immune system, and throws a huge wet blanket on your libido. Active women are half as likely to develop depression and anxiety as their sedentary counterparts. They sleep better at night and feel more energetic and relaxed during the day. And you can get a quality pair of running shoes for the price of one session with a shrink.

You'll drop those final pounds. Exercise helps you reach your weight loss goals. Share those goals with your family, and tell them that you need their help and encouragement in reaching them. That includes pitching in around the house so that you have time to work out. Have a family celebration when you reach your goals.

You can make it a date. You can have fitness as well as social time with girlfriends without taking tons of time for both. Instead of meeting for drinks and dinner, meet to go skating, jogging, or biking, or head to the gym together. You'll be able to chat and catch up on each other's lives, and you'll get your butts in shape as a bonus.

It's great family time. The family that sweats together stays together! Instead of always working out without your man or your kids, take them with you sometimes. Plan a day hike. Do a family run/bike ride. Spend the day swimming and rafting on a lake. The more you do together, the more everyone will appreciate taking active time on their own too.

You can talk to God. Consider it moving meditation. Lots of women use their workout time to get connected to their spiritual self. Hey, it's hard to feel selfish about forgoing mundane tasks such as dishes and laundry for a long run when you know that you're not just training your body but also feeding your soul.

Ten weeks of strength training actually reduced clinical depression symptoms more successfully than standard counseling.

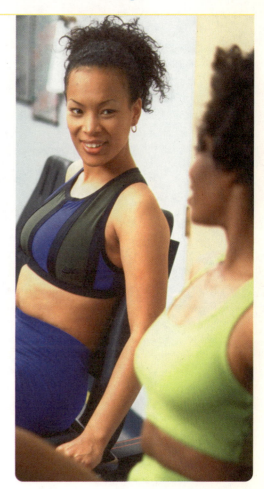

You don't have to leave home. Just *can't* get out of the house? Pick up some dumbbells and workout tapes, and exercise around your kids' school and nap schedules. You won't feel like you're straining the household by leaving for long stretches, but you'll still get in shape.

Exercise makes you interesting. Whether you run, swim, or take yoga classes, working out gives you and your mate (and friends and family) something to talk about. Consider your workouts time spent making you a healthier, happier, and more interesting person.

Time is short! Although it's a subject we avoid while we're young and kicking, our lives won't last forever. Whether you believe we go on to another place, are reborn as turtles, or end up on another planet, this is it for now. Make the most of the body you have, and live your life to the fullest, with no apologies necessary.

It's like brushing your teeth. If you plot out a relatively consistent exercise routine, everyone around you will simply adapt to it and not expect you to be around during those times. That makes it more predictable and less stressful for all involved. If folks still have trouble remembering, post your schedule on a calendar where it can be seen by everyone.

Just do it. People are amazingly adaptable creatures. After the first few weeks of your new exercise regimen, the husband, kids, and boss won't blink an eye at your short absences. And you'll come to realize that they really can manage without you after all—at least for a little while.

Stay Psyched!

Uncover your hidden motivators to keep exercise interesting

Most women can pile a sky-high mountain of excuses for giving up their workouts. Not enough time. Too much work. Family obligations. They're all valid, of course. But what about those high-achieving gals with fast-paced careers, two or three kids, outside hobbies, *and* a consistent exercise routine? The bottom line is that women quit exercising because they're not sufficiently motivated, says exercise researcher Wayne Westcott, PhD.

It's a common problem, which is why creating motivation is an essential part of any training plan.

One very simple, yet very overlooked, way to stay motivated is simply doing exercise you like, says Ross Andersen, PhD, assistant professor of medicine at Johns Hopkins University School of Medicine in Baltimore. To make sure you stick with your routine, you

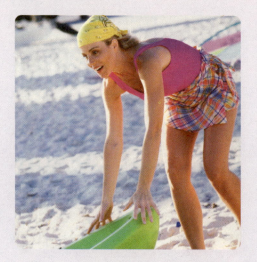

need to find the activity that actually motivates you to exercise. The following quiz will help you match your personal motivations to the right exercises.

CIRCLE ONE ANSWER PER STATEMENT.

1. In my life, I wish I had more:

    a. quiet time.

    b. time with friends or to meet new people.

    c. time outside.

    d. fun "toys."

    e. freedom.

2. I feel happiest when I'm:

    a. curled up with a book.

    b. out dancing.

    c. outside.

    d. spending the day shopping.

    e. at a new restaurant.

3. At a party, I'm most likely to:

    a. talk to my spouse or date.

    b. cut loose and mingle.

    c. take a tour of the house and check out the furnishings and artwork.

    d. go out shopping days before for just the right dress and accessories.

    e. sample everything at the buffet table.

4. My friends would describe me as:
   a. thoughtful.
   b. gregarious.
   c. outdoorsy.
   d. a collector.
   e. pleasure loving.

5. My dream car is a(n):
   a. convertible.
   b. minivan.
   c. SUV.
   d. sports car.
   e. luxury automobile.

Score yourself: Tally up the number of times you circled each letter. The one circled most is your predominant motivator. If you have a fairly even split (i.e., two b's and two d's), try the activities in both of those categories. If you have one of each, you have some experimenting to do, but that's half the fun!

IF YOU CIRCLED ...

MOSTLY A'S
   You are motivated by: Time for yourself. You appreciate relaxing with your own thoughts and having quiet, stress-free time to enjoy and contemplate life.
   For exercise: Try stress-reducing solitary exercises such as yoga, walking, running, swimming, hiking, or strength training with home exercise equipment.

MOSTLY B'S
   You are motivated by: Social interaction. You thrive when you're in large groups. You love to meet new people and try new things—the more the merrier!
   For exercise: Try fun social activities such as working out at a large neighborhood gym, taking group exercise classes, or participating in walking/hiking clubs, tennis, or team sports such as volleyball.

MOSTLY C'S
   You are motivated by: The great outdoors. You love the beauty of nature, seeing new places, and taking in the world at large.

You're in your glory when tending your flower beds and herb boxes or strolling through a new park.
   For exercise: Try outdoor sporting activities such as hiking, sea kayaking or canoeing, mountain biking, or walking.

MOSTLY D'S
   You are motivated by: New fun gear to try. You're like a kid on Christmas morning every time you get a new "toy" to try out. You love to shop and check out all the interesting stuff.
   For exercise: Try gear-oriented activities such as golf, bicycling, or cross-country skiing, buy some home exercise equipment, or try racquet sports such as tennis or squash.

MOSTLY E'S
   You are motivated by: Pleasure and rewards. You want palpable results for your efforts. You enjoy dining out and treating yourself to nights on the town.
   For exercise: Try quick-result, calorie-burning activities such as strength training, stairclimbing, jumping rope, power walking, or jogging.

CHAPTER 22

10 Gotta-Have Workout Toys

New exercise gadgets can be fun, motivational, and may even help keep you safe

No matter how much you love your fitness regime, there's nothing like a cool new gizmo to freshen up your exercise sessions. (Just think about how much more exciting jumping became once the pogo stick was introduced!) Here are 10 gotta-have gadgets that can make your workouts more effective, more pleasant, and more satisfying—without costing you an arm and a leg.

A fun way to round out your exercise program.

1. Get a Jump on Fitness

Jumping rope is a superquick and easy way to build bone and blast fat. Track the calories you burn while you jump with HealthyJump, a smart jump rope from Tanita that counts your jumps and calories burned. It's fully adjustable, a cinch to program, and has comfy, ergonomic grips. HealthyJump is available in major sporting goods stores for $19.99. Visit the Tanita Corporation of America's Web site at www.tanitascale.com/healthyjump.html.

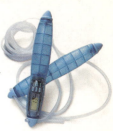

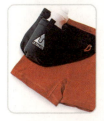

2. Wear Your Water

You need to stay hydrated during those long power walks or day hikes. Carrying water can be a drag, but not so with the Walker's WaterPack by Ultimate Direction. This adjustable pack carries a 20-oz bottle and has two zippered pockets for keys, snacks, and a stash of spare cash. Cost: $28. Available at www.walkerswarehouse.com.

3. Walk and Rock

Studies show that music can help you walk or run longer and faster while making the exertion feel more effortless. Working out to music is easier than ever with the TuneBelt CD or Cassette Holder. It's comfortable, bounce-free, and reflective. CD $24, cassette $22. Available at www.walkerswarehouse.com.

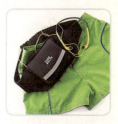

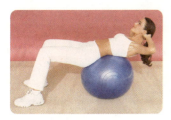

4. Have a Ball!

Americans spend more than $200 million a year on abdominal devices in a quest for flat, firm abs—but most of these products are ineffective or even dangerous. For a real ab toner, pick up an inflatable exercise ball. Crunches on an exercise ball are much more effective than doing them on the floor. And they feel better too. Exercise balls are available in most major sporting goods stores and cost around $30. Or visit www.walkerswarehouse.com.

5. Put Your Best Foot Forward

When sore feet have you down, pick up *Hands on Feet* (Running Press, 2001) by Michelle R. Kluck, an easy-to-follow guide that explains how to give relaxing and therapeutic foot massage. It makes a perfect gift for that special foot rubber in your life! The book even comes with a pair of socks illustrated on the bottom to show what areas of the soles correspond to each part of the body, so you can target any problem areas. Available wherever books are sold. Cost: $14.

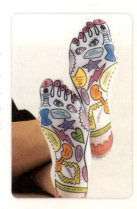

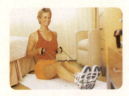

6. Tone Up with Tubing

Exercise bands, or tubing, are superlight, portable, take-anywhere fitness equipment. They're a must-have for every busy woman. Just pack and go to do rows, biceps curls, lateral raises, squats, and much more on the road. Cost: about $6. Check out the Spri Products Web site at www.spriproducts.com.

7. Make Every Step Count

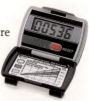

Fitness researchers recommend taking 10,000 steps a day for optimum health. But if you're not careful, time at the desk can shave your step count in half, if not more. Keep yourself on track with the *Prevention* Digital Step Pedometer. It's easy to use, lightweight, and has a convenient waist clip. Cost: $26.95. Available at www.walkerswarehouse.com.

8. Keep Moving—Pain-Free

Foot pain can bring your exercise program to a screeching halt, and it affects a whopping 75% of Americans at some point in their life. For some people, orthotics (shoe inserts) may be the answer. Orthotics can provide extra cushioning, take pressure off common sore spots such as your heel or the ball of your foot, and even help control the motion of your feet as you move. Try Dr. Scholl's Advantage Sport. Cost: $14. Available at major drugstores.

9. Roll with It

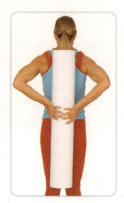

Biofoam rollers (firm Styrofoam cylinders) are a great way to strengthen your core muscles and improve your balance. They can also relieve nagging back pain by strengthening the trunk muscles that stabilize your spine. Try this move: With your feet flat on the floor, lie back on a Biofoam roller extended along your spine from your butt to your neck. Raise your arms straight up so your hands point toward the ceiling. Lift your right foot off the floor. Slowly move your arms to the right until they are almost parallel to the floor, then move them to the other side. Bring your arms back to center. Then switch legs, and repeat; continue switching sides for 10 minutes. Do this move once or twice daily. To get a 3-foot-long, 6-inch-round Biofoam roller, check out Perform Better's Web site at www.performbetter.com. Cost: $16.95.

10. Stay Safe in the Sun

Sunscreen with an SPF of 15 or higher can protect you from skin cancer. But you need to reapply it every 2 hours for maximum protection, something few of us do when we're on the go. Sunbuddy makes sun safety a no-brainer. These single-use packets provide a palmful of sunscreen for full-body coverage. Choose from five waterproof varieties, including insect repellent and made-for-babies formulas. Cost: $1 a packet. For buying info, go to www.sunbuddy.com.

CHAPTER 23

Workouts to Match Your Mood

Don't let your emotional ups and downs sabotage your fitness

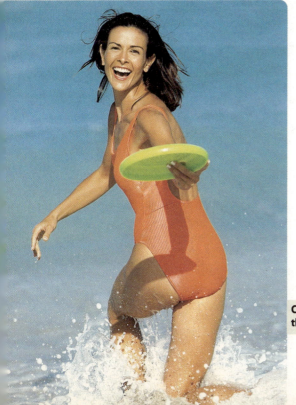

Cut loose from the old routine.

You may love your urban rhythms funk class. But let's face it, getting psyched up to shake your boo-tay can be pretty tough when another round of pink slips has fallen at your job or your boyfriend was AWOL last weekend. Here's how to get fit even when you don't feel like exercising.

Are you stale?

There's nothing like the first few months of an exercise routine. You're losing fat, gaining tone, and enjoying the payoff of sticking to your program as you zip up those jeans you haven't worn in a while. But when that routine starts becoming *routine*, all that progress can come to a screeching halt as you hit what's commonly known as "the plateau." The solution: Keep things interesting. If you recognize yourself in the list below, it's time to try something new.

10 signs it's time to change your exercise routine.

1. You skip your workouts to bathe the cat.

2. You own one exercise outfit, but you only need to wash it every 2 weeks.

3. Your hair looks as good at the end of your workout as it did before you started.

4. The last time you changed your routine was during the Bush administration—the first one.

5. You still exercise to Olivia Newton-John's "Physical."

6. Of the 24 machines at your gym, 23 of them are a complete mystery to you.

7. The instructor on your favorite exercise video now lags behind you.

8. You think crunches are the funny noises your knees make.

9. You've broken the snooze button on the alarm you set for early morning workouts.

10. You think Pilates is a new restaurant in New York City.

"Lots of people skip working out when their mood isn't ideal because they don't have the mental energy to switch gears," says mental health and exercise expert Jack Raglin, PhD, of Indiana University. "But the trick lies in finding the right workout to match the mood you're in." For example, some workouts have a calming effect, while others are stimulating. Here's what Dr. Raglin recommends to keep you exercising no matter what your state of mind.

Down with the blues? "Studies have shown that even mild exercise, about 40% of your max heart rate, can lift your mood," says Dr. Raglin. "So if you're not up for the usual high-energy stuff, do some leisure activity you enjoy, such as digging in your flower beds, hiking with your dog, or walking in a park. View it as mental recreation, not exercise."

Steaming mad? "As tempting as it may be, skip the kickboxing," he advises. "You can't punch away anger. Instead, do something that involves your mind and keeps you from focusing and ruminating on what has you angry. Play racquetball, or take that hip new aerobics class you've been wanting to try. Learning new moves will free your mind from what's been upsetting you."

Bored out of your skull? "Being around people is a quick and easy way to beat boredom. Playing a sport with them is even better," says Dr. Raglin. "Try some tennis or golf. Get together with a group that walks, jogs, or goes for bike rides on a regular basis. Play soccer or shoot hoops with your kids. Being outside with other people is invigorating and engages your mind."

Stressed to the max? "When your brain is overwhelmed and anxious, you need to turn to a mindless activity to settle it down. Something repetitive such as swimming, cycling, or walking on a treadmill requires little mental input and is most effective at reducing feelings of stress and increasing calmness," he says.

"You can't punch away anger. Instead, do something that involves your mind and keeps you from focusing and ruminating on what has you angry." —Jack Raglin, PhD

Walking on sunshine? A happy mood can sideline a workout as easily as a sad one, especially if you feel too "up" to do your same old routine. "Take advantage of good moods to go out and challenge yourself. See if you can run 1 more mile than usual, or add another set to your weight routine. Use that energy to feel even better," advises Dr. Raglin.

Never in the Mood?

If your workout's feeling like too much work no matter what you do, it might be more of a physical problem than an emotional one. Fatigue during exercise stems from a number of physical and psychological reasons, but usually it's an easy fix. Try these tips to stop the energy drain.

Pump iron. Iron is essential for high energy levels. Make sure your diet includes 18 mg a day by eating lean meats, legumes, leafy greens, and whole grains. Include citrus fruit and juice with vitamin C, which improves iron absorption.

Fuel up early. Eating the bulk of your calories in the early part of the day will give you the energy you need to make it through daytime workouts. Many women on weight loss plans find it easier to eat less during the day and more at night—exactly the

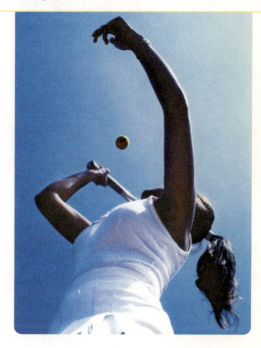

opposite plan for optimal energy and weight loss.

Wet your whistle. Dehydration can seriously drag your energy down. Research shows that even when you drink eight glasses of water a day, 45 minutes of exercise can put you into a dehydrated state. Don't rely on thirst as a measure of need—to prevent exercise fatigue, take a sip of water every 15 to 20 minutes while you work out.

Snack first. One small study showed that cyclists who had eaten a small meal before their workouts lasted 30 minutes longer than those with empty stomachs. Try yogurt, a banana, or some graham crackers to keep your energy high.

FIT TIP!

Be a quick change artist

If you don't have the time or opportunity to do something new, alter your usual workout. Take your run outside for a change of scenery. Hike through the park. Try a different class or machine at the gym. Let your mood be your guide.

bonus beauty section!

170 **Get Glowing from Head to Toe**
A no-fail regimen for rejuvenating
your on-the-go skin

176 **Crowning Glory: Here's to Hair!**
The right cut, color, and style can carry you
from flabby to fabulous

180 **Dress for Exercise Success**
This activewear will keep you going
and going and going!

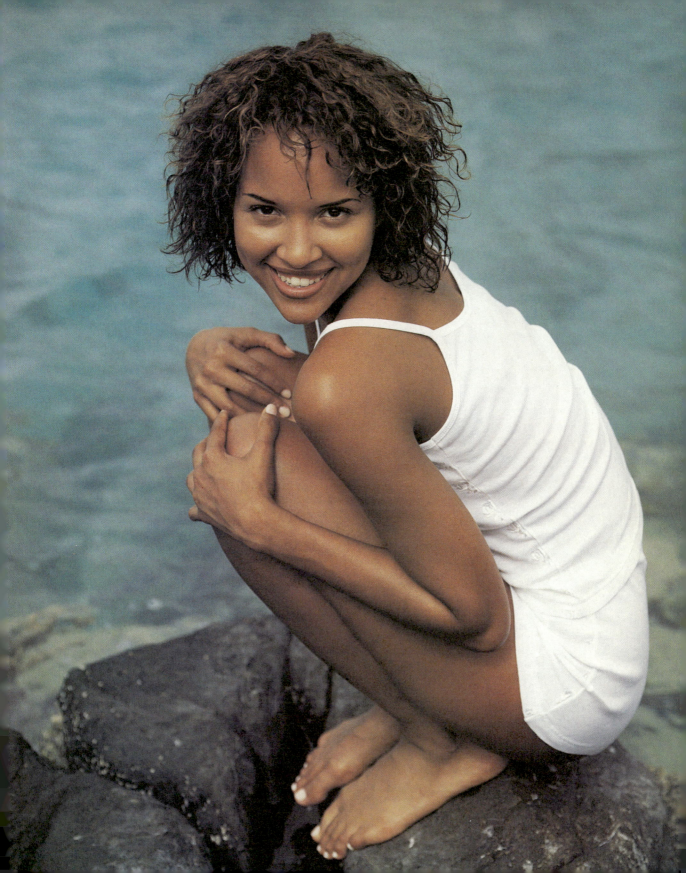

Get Glowing from Head to Toe

A no-fail regimen for rejuvenating your on-the-go skin

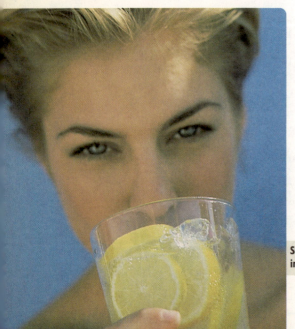

Running, skiing, biking, and salsa dancing are great for your body and soul, but all that sun, sweat, and wind can be rough on your skin. Cosmetics companies have developed hundreds of products for protecting and preserving the skin. A few may even reverse some of the visible signs of aging, such as wrinkles and age spots. But before reaching for specific skin care products, keep in mind that your skin reflects your life. You need to include both product and lifestyle for healthy, glowing skin.

Skintastic—from the inside out.

Everyday Skin Smarts

If you smoke, bake in the sun for a tan, eat junk food, gain too much weight, or experience a lot of stress, your skin will pay for it. If, on the other hand, you relax often, eat healthful meals, and generally maintain positive lifestyle habits, you'll be rewarded with skin that's smooth and firm, even in your later years. Here are a few healthy-glow steps that skin-savvy gals should follow each day.

Heap on the H₂0. You need at least eight glasses of water daily to keep the cells of your skin plump, making them look smoother and younger, says Kathy A. Fields, MD, clinical instructor of dermatology at the University of California, San Francisco. Equally important to making the skin look plump, she adds, is good humidity in the air around you. Consider running a humidifier during cold, dry winter months.

Screen out the sun. Sunscreen is the only way to prevent future skin damage because it blocks the sun's ultraviolet radiation. Sun exposure also accounts for about 90% of all skin cancers. Doctors advise applying sunscreen lavishly after your moisturizer but at least 30 minutes prior to sun exposure, then reapply every 2 hours.

DO JUST ONE THING!

Milk it!

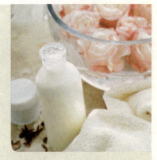

If you try no other skin care product, try one of the many new moisturizers containing milk. Milk as a beauty agent has been around for centuries. (Think Cleopatra and her milk baths.) For years, dermatologists have prescribed milk compresses to soothe inflamed, sunburned, or irritated skin. Now, milk-based skin care is becoming more popular. Though there's no real scientific evidence available to tell us *why* it's good for the skin, there are plenty of good reasons to try it. Milk proteins such as whey (the watery substance you get when you separate the curds from the milk) and various other milk ingredients are helpful for good skin health. They work to moisturize the skin. An added bonus: Milk will reduce redness and inflammation when applied to the skin.

The women who will benefit most from "milking" their skin are those with sensitive skin, or skin that is prone to extreme dryness due to temperature changes or windburn. Women who suffer from a skin condition such as rosacea will also benefit from using milk-based products. When buying, look for ingredients such as milk protein, milk lipids, or whey. And don't try pulling a Cleopatra and actually bathing in milk or applying it straight from the carton. Milk is made up of mostly water, which evaporates as the milk dries. This will actually dry out your skin. Milk also spoils very quickly, and when it does, it smells bad! Finally, cosmetic milk is highly concentrated. You'd need an awful lot of store-bought milk to get the same effect.

Choose products that block both UVA and UVB rays and that have an SPF of at least 15.

Butt out. Smoking ages your skin—and fast—by constricting bloodflow, causing your skin to lose out on valuable nutrients. Quitting now will help spare your skin years down the road.

Follow a regimen. Pamper your skin with a daily cleansing and moisturizing regimen. In the past few years, cosmetics companies have created rejuvenating products that really can protect the skin, reverse wrinkles, and generally make you look younger. The six-step process that follows is a great place to start.

6 Steps to Young Skin

Follow the regimen below, and you'll always be putting your best face forward.

STEP 1: LATHER UP.

Skin needs to be clean to be healthy, so it's important to use cleansers to gently wash away dust, makeup, and surface oils. Use nonsoap cleansers; they're much less drying than regular soaps. David J. Leffell, MD, chief of dermatologic surgery at Yale University School of Medicine, recommends Neutrogena Extra Gentle Cleanser, Aquanil, or Cetaphil.

Consider an exfoliating cleanser if you're over 40. The skin naturally sheds its top layer, uncovering the fresh, youthful-looking layer underneath. In women under 40, this shedding occurs every 30 days. After 40, it slows to every 60 days, which makes the skin dry, the pores clogged and enlarged, and the complexion dull and sallow. You can speed up the process by using a scrub soap that contains tiny polyethylene beads, which gently remove dead cells and moisturize the skin. Don't bother with scrub soaps that contain pits from almonds or walnuts, Dr. Fields advises. They

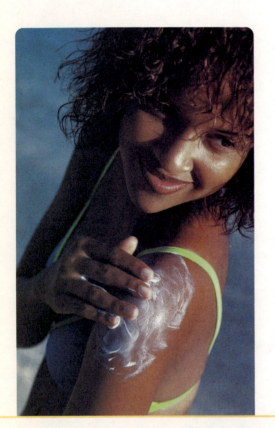

If you relax often, eat healthful meals, and generally maintain positive lifestyle habits, you'll be rewarded with skin that's smooth and firm, even in your later years.

can actually damage the skin. If you're 40 or older, you can use gentle scrub soaps every day, says Dr. Fields. If you're under 40, use them only once a week or as needed.

STEP 2: **MOISTURIZE.**

Moisturizers hydrate and plump up the cells on the skin's surface, which makes the skin softer. Use oil-free products; they contain an ingredient called dimethicone. It's a type of silicone that gives moisturizers a light feel, Dr. Fields says. A good example would be Oil of Olay.

Keep your moisturizers simple. If you have sensitive skin, avoid moisturizers loaded with fragrances and extracts. Check the label: It should list fewer than 10 ingredients, says Dr. Fields. Cetaphil is a good choice as a moisturizer for sensitive skin, as well as Eucerin and Almay products.

Moisturize after showers or baths. The moisturizer will form a barrier over the moisture that's already on your skin, which gives it time to be absorbed by the cells, says Dr. Leffell.

STEP 3: **SMOOTH OUT WRINKLES.**

Many anti-aging products claim to "erase" wrinkles and make the skin look years younger. Some of this is marketing hype, but there's good evidence that products that contain natural acids (alpha or beta hydroxy acids) really can erase fine lines or brown spots, at least temporarily. They work by exfoliating the superficial layers of skin and can actually stimulate collagen production, which plumps up the skin and makes it look softer and fresher, says Lisa Kates, MD, a dermatologist at Cook County Hospital in Chicago.

Alpha hydroxy acids come in moisturizers, eye creams, and many other products. Terms to

Vitamin Lotions: Hip or Hype?

Everything from moisturizers to mascara contains vitamins these days. Some have well-documented benefits, while others are just expensive additives. Here are the real skin-savers.

➤ **Vitamin A.** Found in products such as Retin-A, vitamin A increases cell turnover, lightens freckles and age spots, and gives skin a more even tone and texture. Can be irritating to sensitive skin.

➤ **Vitamin B.** Vitamin B_3 (niacin) has long been used in Asian skin care products as a whitener and brightener.

➤ **Vitamin C.** Topical vitamin C (L-ascorbic acid) functions as an antioxidant, helping to protect the skin against damage from free radicals.

➤ **Vitamin D.** This vitamin helps regulate cell reproduction and turnover and is routinely used to treat psoriasis. May not help normal skin.

➤ **Vitamin F.** This is linoleic acid. It probably soothes skin when topically applied, but it's not proven.

➤ **Vitamin K.** This vitamin helps bruises fade faster. It also inhibits melanin production and, with continued use, can minimize the appearance of dark undereye circles.

look for on labels include glycolic acid (derived from sugarcane), lactic acid (from milk), tartaric acid (from grapes), citric acid (from citrus fruits), malic acid (from apples), and mandelic acid (from walnuts). You may want to look for products that contain salicylic acid, which is a beta hydroxy acid. In women with sensitive skin, some of these products can be irritating. It's essential to use a sunscreen and avoid excessive sun exposure when using these products, because they increase your sensitivity to the sun. And be patient: It may take 6 to 8 weeks to see a difference.

STEP 4: FADE THOSE SPOTS.

After decades of sun exposure, nearly everyone will develop pigment-related problems, such as age spots or freckles. It isn't always possible to eliminate them completely, but they can almost always be faded to the point of invisibility with bleaching creams. These products contain active ingredients such as hydroquinone or kojic acid, which interfere with pigment formation, Dr. Kates says. Kojic acid is found in Nu Skin Skin-Brightening Complex and other products. For the most part, it doesn't work as well as hydroquinone.

Prescription-strength hydroquinone tends to give better results than over-the-counter (OTC) products and can be used with OTC products that contain kojic acid. Use daily or twice a day as tolerated, and avoid the sun; otherwise, the brown spots and age spots will return within hours.

STEP 5: FRESHEN UP WITH MASKS OR PEELS.

Masks leave your face feeling clean and refreshed. Peels are somewhat different. They remove the top layer of skin and lighten some brown spots.

When you're shopping for mask products at the cosmetics counter, it's important to find one that matches your skin type. If you have dry skin, buy a hydrating mask. For oily skin, use clay masks or "deep cleansers." For acne, use a sulfur or "purifying" mask.

If you want something stronger, go for a glycolic acid peel. Performed by dermatologists, this is sometimes called the "lunchtime peel" because it works so quickly. The dermatologist will apply glycolic acid to your face, and it goes to work removing dead cells and quickly uncovers the younger, smoother skin underneath. The peel tin-

Glow Like a Pro

Who knows better about healthy, shimmery skin than a dermatologist? We asked Leslie Baumann, MD, director of cosmetic dermatology at the University of Miami Cosmetic Center, how she keeps her skin looking so young. Here's what works for her.

"I use Retin-A at night, and Eucerin Q10 Anti-Wrinkle Sensitive Skin facial moisturizer underneath my sunscreen. Eucerin's active ingredient, coenzyme Q10, is an antioxidant. There haven't been enough solid studies to show whether it offers real benefits topically. Still, I love how it feels as a moisturizer."

After decades of sun exposure, nearly everyone will develop pigment-related problems, such as age spots or freckles . . . they can almost always be faded to the point of invisibility.

gles, but it isn't uncomfortable, says Seth L. Matarasso, MD, associate clinical professor of dermatology at the University of California, San Francisco, and a dermatologist in San Francisco. Peels cost between $75 and $150, and you can get them as often as once a month.

STEP 6: SAY GOODBYE TO PUFFY EYES.

Few things can make you look more tired (or older) than puffy eyes. They're usually caused by such things as fatigue, water retention, allergies, or even a reaction to eye makeup. To quickly tighten the skin and help your eyes look younger, here's what experts advise.

Reduce puffiness with tea bags. Brew a cup of tea using two tea bags. Set the bags aside until they're cool, then place them on the puffy areas of your eyes for a few minutes. The cool moisture can reduce swelling for up to 24 hours. In addition, tea contains tannins, compounds that reduce eye inflammation, says Dr. Matarasso. You can get similar effects by placing cool cucumber slices or even cooled spoons on the puffy areas, he adds.

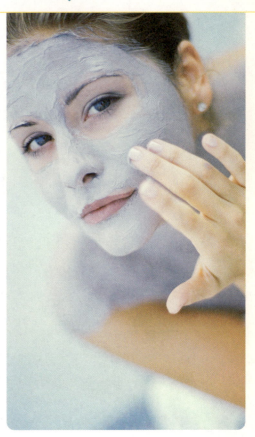

CHAPTER 25

Crowning Glory: Here's to Hair!

The right cut, color, and style can carry you from flabby to fabulous

Getting the right hairstyle can do more than give you a vibrant, attractive reflection in the mirror. It can be a way to express yourself too. There's no better time to try out a new "do" than after losing some weight and getting in shape; it sends the message that you feel more confident, daring, and self-assured. Heck, even if you haven't lost all the weight you want, you can still feel fabulous after a trip to the hairstylist. Changing your hair cut, color, or style can pave the way for creating a whole new you. So book an appointment today. If you're not happy with your current stylist, get a referral from your friend with the best-dressed tresses. A new you is waiting!

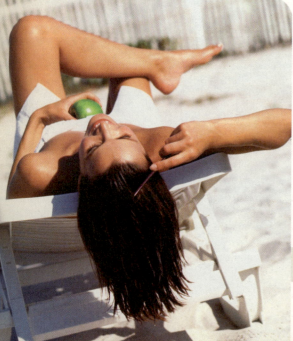

Be the mane event with a new style.

A Cut to Complement Your Body

Too often, women find that their hair looks great in the bathroom mirror, but when they back up and look at their hair *and* their body, they just don't match.

"I think the reason people get the wrong haircut is because stylists sit them down, cover up their bodies, and try to fix some sort of problem with the face," says Laurie Krauz, an image consultant in New York City. She suggests that you look at the whole picture instead.

Stand tall. Your height should play a role in how you wear your hair. If you're short, don't wear your hair very long. You'll only look shorter if your hair covers up your neck and body, says Nick Berardi, senior creative director at Vidal Sassoon in New York City.

Trust your lines. Let your hairstyle complement the shape of your body. Check a full-length mirror to gauge your body's lines, Krauz says. When you look at yourself head-on, is the line that starts from under your shoulder and extends to your hip straight or curvy? Are your arms and legs angular or soft? If you have a straight body, get an angular, blunt cut. If your body is curvy, let your hair look soft and flowing.

Give your hair a little height. A little height and width can make all the difference when you're trying to balance out a not-so-small body. "If you wear your hair flat or straight around your face, you'll look heavier," says Kenneth Battelle, owner and master stylist of Kenneth's Salon in New York City. Watch out for super-short haircuts too. "The shorter it is, the heavier you look," he adds.

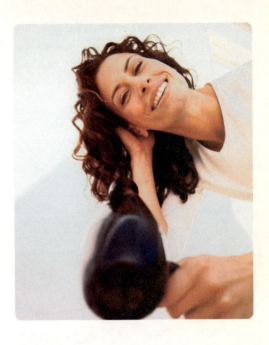

Face Facts

While body shape is important when choosing a new style, don't forget to consider the shape of your face too. When you create a balance between your face, body, and hair, you let people know that you're in charge and in style. Take some advice from the experts on how to achieve the look you want.

Take a measure. The key to looking great is proportion, according to Catherine Schuller, fashion retail editor of *Mode* magazine and author of *The Ultimate Plus-Size Modeling Guide*. While hair with a little height is important for balancing

FIT TIP! **Watch falling hair**

If your hair is thinning, suspect a hormone connection such as low estrogen levels or hypothyroidism (an underactive thyroid gland). See your doctor if you're experiencing unexplained loss of locks.

out a fuller-figured body, make sure that you add height in proportion to your face and overall size. Don't get the height you need by teasing either. Instead, add texture and volume with layers for a softer, easier lift at the crown.

While standing in half-profile to your mirror, measure the distance from the bottom of your chin to the top of your ear. Then measure the distance from the top of your ear to the top of your hair. Both measurements should be the same. If your hair is higher, take it down to match the distance from chin to ear.

DO JUST ONE THING!

Hydrate frazzled hair

Sun, surf, sweat, wind, and winter can leave your hair dry as sand in the Sahara. Revive dry locks with flower and plant power. The following products are some of our favorites.

Intense Moisturizer

Apricot and wild cherry shampoo and deep conditioner work together to hydrate dry, brittle hair. **Truly, Madly, Deeply by Freeman** is available at drugstores and mass market retailers everywhere. Visit the Freeman Web site at www.freemancosmetics.com. ($3.29)

Vitality Blast

Give your hair a little CPR with a 10-minute intensive treatment chock-full of herbs and vitamins. **Lifetex Wellness Vitality Blasts by Wella** are available in two formulations. Call toll-free (866) LIFETEX (543-3839), or go online at www.lifetexwellness.com to find an outlet near you. ($14.99)

Soothing Trio

This jasmine and lavender shampoo, conditioner, and moisturizing treatment makes hair feel soft and healthy. **BIO by Bath and Body Works** is available in six formulations. To find a Bath and Body Works store near you, call (800) 395-1001 (US only). ($7.50–$8)

Curl Care

This moisturizing trio defines curls and smoothes out frizz. **L'Oreal Curl VIVE** shampoos, conditioners, and spray gels are available at retailers across the US. Check out the L'Oreal Web site at www.loreal.com. ($3.69 each)

High Shine

You'll love the way **Aveda's Purefum Brilliant Humectant Pomade** moisturizes hair and tames flyaways. Aloe, sea kelp, and flaxseed give hair that polished look. And it smells clean and fresh. To find a salon near you, call (800) 328-0849; in Canada, call (800) 689-1066; or go online at www.aveda.com. ($12)

Too often, women find that their hair looks great in the bathroom mirror, but when they back up and look at their hair *and* their body, they just don't match.

Notice the shape of things. By breaking your look down into shapes, you can create balance. "I'm like an artist playing with shapes and trying to make sense out of them," says Richard Cordoba, a hair care specialist at Sam Wong Hair Salon in New York City. When you put different shapes together on yourself, some things are going to feel more balanced than others, he says.

An oval face is the easiest to work with because most shapes look good on it, Cordoba says. But keep in mind that long, straight hair will make an oval face look too long. To complement this shape, get your hair cut in layers, especially around your face.

But if your jaw is wide, put a round shape on your style. Don't put a bob line at the jaw because it will accentuate your jaw's square shape, Berardi says. Instead, add bangs and layers that start at the cheekbone and go down to give your face a round frame that will offset your jaw, Cordoba says.

And if your face is round, complement it with a longer, layered cut. Keep your hair one length in the back, and put layers around your face that start either at your cheekbone or jawline and go down. Remember that long hair makes your face look longer, and rounder cuts make your face look rounder.

Color to Dye For

Now that you have the right style, it's time to think shade. Maybe you're covering those wiry white strands, or you're just bored with your natural hue. Whatever the case, a little touch-up can brighten your entire look. Here are a few cardinal rules of getting color.

Go back in time. The best way to look younger is to choose a shade that is a little lighter than what you had when you were a kid, according to Brad Johns, artistic director of the Avon Centre in New York City. "The lighter you go, as long as you don't get too white, the more youthful the appearance." If you were dark brown as a kid, choose medium brown. If you were light brown, choose dark blonde. And if you were blonde, stay blonde.

Make it multicolor. Get your hair fully colored, then put highlights near your face. Stick with lighter and warmer colors for a youthful look. A dark frame around your face will only make you look older because the dark hair throws shadows that define lines.

CHAPTER 26

Dress for Exercise Success

This activewear will keep you going and going and going!

Workout clothes have evolved light years from frumpy gray sweats (hallelujah!) and colored tights with thong body suits (double hallelujah!). Today's active-wear is so comfy and stylish that you can go from the bike trail to the coffee shop without a cover-up or a change of clothes. Here are some of our favorites that will keep you looking and feeling your best.

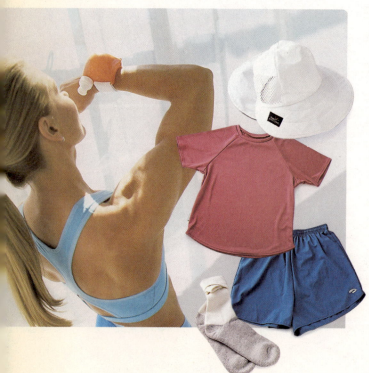

Sweat never had such style!

Swingin' Skorts

Sports skorts are a fun, flattering addition to your workout wardrobe. Underneath a flirty-looking skirted front are practical, comfortable athletic shorts. Made from nonwrinkling soft polyester and nylon Lycra, these skirted wonders offer super comfort and full coverage. And sportswear manufacturer Terry Precision Cycling offers a special skort to match most everything you do. Are you a cyclist who loves the comfort of padded spandex bike shorts but hates the look? The bike Commuter skort ($80) has a padded seat. Tennis, anyone? The Swinger ($75) features a convenient ball pocket. And the Traveler ($38) is a slightly longer skort with 8-inch athletic shorts and hidden pockets on the side, front compartment, and rear hip; it's ideal for walking, hiking, or golfing. To order, call Terry Precision Cycling at (800) 289-8379, or visit their Web site at www. terrybicycles.com.

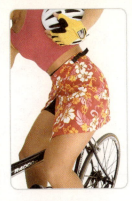

Smart Undies

Those lumpy, frumpy cotton long johns of yesteryear were undeniably great to sleep in. But today's long underwear are designed with smart fiber technology that will keep you warm and dry in even the nastiest weather. They're also soft and sleek and feel downright sexy—even under jeans.

Here are our three favorites. They're available at sporting goods stores, or contact the manufacturers for more info.

➤ **Columbia's Titanium Outlast** technical base layers automatically regulate your body temperature. So if you're too hot, your body heat is transferred outward; but if you're cold, this performance material "knows" to trap body heat. Call (800) 622-6953, or check www.columbia.com for buying information. ($65 top, $65 pant)

➤ **REI's Midweight MTS** base layers have a compound inside the material that kills odor-causing bacteria. The result: You smell fresh all day long. For catalog sales, call (800) 426-4840, or check www.rei.com. ($28 top, $28 pant)

➤ **Brooks Runderwear** feels silky smooth and is supercomfortable. The polyester fabrics wick moisture away from your skin, and mesh panels let your body breathe, so you don't get overheated. Call (800) 2-BROOKS (227-6657), or check www.brooksrunning.com for buying information. ($26 top, $26 pant)

Sock It to It!

Nothing wrecks a good workout faster than a bad blister. And the easiest way to prevent blisters, as well as sweaty, sore feet, is with quality socks. Here are some of our favorites.

FOR HOT WORKOUTS.

When the heat is on, the right socks can keep you cool.

➤ **DeFeet's Cush Aireator** is thin and oh-so-breathable. Cost is $14. To locate a dealer, call (800) 688-3067, or visit their Web site at www.defeet.com.

These cool treats make summer workouts more fun

Heat and humidity putting a damper on your fitness plans? Here are five workout essentials to keep you feeling fresh even when the heat's on high.

➤ **HYDROSPORT WRIST WATER BOTTLES.** An easy way to stay hydrated: Carry 4 oz of water in a small bottle that attaches to your wrist; take a sip every 10 minutes. $15

➤ **EXPEDITION SPORTHAT.** A full brim and rear veil protect your face and neck from the sun. Mesh side panels offer excellent ventilation, and an internal sweatband soaks up perspiration. $35

➤ **BROOKS SILC TEE.** Enjoy the silky feel of this ultralight shirt that also wicks moisture. $36.95

➤ **BROOKS POWERPRO SPORTS BRA.** Comfort and support in a featherlight, supersoft bra that's quick drying and won't chafe tender underarms. $34

➤ **BROOKS MICRO-POLY PACERS.** No more chafing: These shorts are ultralightweight and made for motion. Available in a rainbow of colors. $34.95

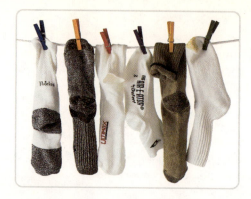

➤ **GoldToe Coolmax Cotton Crew** is also silky thin to keep you cool. Two pairs cost $9. Available in department stores, call (800) 523-8265, or go online at www.goldtoe.com.

➤ **X-Static Socks** feature silver-coated nylon threads that act as natural antibacterial agents to fight odor. They're great at wicking moisture too. Go to www.walkerswarehouse.com to get a three-pack for $19.99. Or call toll-free (888) 972-9255.

FOR OVER-40 FEET.

As you get older, you lose the protective fat pads on your feet, but these socks can make up for that loss.

➤ **Thorlo's Lite Walking Crew (LWXW-10)** offers protection and comfort without added bulk and warmth. Cost is $11.99. Call toll-free (888) 846-7567 to find a retailer near you, or visit their Web site at www.thorlo.com.

➤ **Wigwam's Ultimax Performance Walking Crew** has great cushioning and very little bulk. These socks fit great and are super at wicking away sweat. Cost is $8. To order, call (800) 628-5821, or go online at www.wigwam.com.

FOR HIKERS.

Treading all day on rocky trails demands strong, supercomfortable socks such as these.

➤ **Woolrich Lightweight TechnoWool Hiking Socks** feature a special blend that offers the benefits of wool (insulation, durability, and breathability) without the itchiness. They look great too. Cost is $16. To find a retailer, call (800) 995-1299, or visit their Web site at www.woolrich.com.

➤ **Mephisto** hiking socks keep feet blister-free and comfortable no matter what the temperature. Prices range from $10 to $19. Call toll-free (866) 952-7263 for a store directory, or go online at www.mephisto.com.

Great Kicks!

Whether you're walking a marathon or strolling the mall, you've got to have the right shoes. Here are some that will help you put your best foot forward while you walk off the weight.

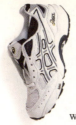

➤ **Asics Gel Tech Walker III** is so comfortable that you can wear them all day long to run errands as well as take a brisk walk. Cost is $85. For more info, call (800) 227-6657, or go to www.brookssports.com.

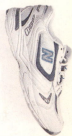

➤ **New Balance 655** is a very comfortable and long-lasting ride with great heel-to-toe motion and stability. Cost is $70. For more info, call (800) 253-7463, or visit www.newbalance.com.

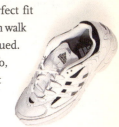

➤ **New Balance 743** is a perfect off-road walking shoe that smoothes out rocks and bumps like you're walking on air. Also provides great traction. Cost is $80. For more info, call (800) 253-7463, or go to www.newbalance.com.

➤ **Nike Air Durham Plus** is a cushiony running shoe that offers plenty of toe room in front, yet hugs your heels in back. Cost is $100. For more info, call (800) 344-6453, or visit www.nike.com.

➤ **Adidas Salus** provides a perfect fit and wonderful feel, so you can walk faster without feeling fatigued. Cost is $65. For more info, call (800) 423-4327, or visit www.adidas.com.

All products are available from The Walker's Warehouse at www.walkerswarehouse.com. Or call toll-free (888) 972-9255.

photo credits

Steve Cole/Getty Images: page 162

Color Day Production/Getty Images: page 167

Color Stock/Getty Images: page 56

Corel Images: page 100

Digital Vision: pages 169, 172

Digital Vision/Getty Images: page 62

Dynamic Graphics: page 32

EyeWire: page 5

Brian Hagiwara/Foodpix: pages 113, 136, 140

John Hamel/Rodale Images: page 156

Hilmar: pages viii, x, xii, 1, 8, 9, 10, 11, 13, 14, 15, 18 (ballerina), 19, 20, 21, 22, 23, 24, 25, 28, 29, 30, 31, 33, 34 (woman stretching), 37 (ball crunch), 40, 42, 47, 48, 51, 53, 54, 60, 74, 75, 76, 77, 78, 80, 81, 82, 83, 85, 104, 107, 109, 157, 160, 163 (ball crunch), 164 (women), 165, 170, 176, 177, 180, 181

Lisa Koenig/Stockfood: page 134

Mitch Mandel/Rodale Images: pages vi, 6, 7, 16, 17, 18 (spine stretch), 30 (woman on step bench), 34, 35, 36, 37, 44, 45, 68, 69, 70, 71, 92, 94 (cereal), 111, 112, 114, 115, 116, 117, 122, 123 (recipe), 124, 125, 126, 127, 129, 130, 131, 132, 133, 135, 137, 138, 139, 140, 141, 142, 143, 144, 145, 148, 149, 151, 152, 153, 159

Neo Vision/Photonica: page 3

Paul Poplis/Foodpix: page 147

Photodisc Collection/Getty Images: page 175

Push/Foodpix: page 146

Rodale Images: pages 95 (pretzel), 120

Martina Sandlkuehler/Jump: page 52

Stockbyte: pages viii, 4, 12, 65, 66, 72, 79, 95 (grapes and tomatoes), 110

Veer: page 171

Christiane Vey/Jump : pages vi, 26, 39

Kurt Wilson/Rodale Images: pages x, 86, 88, 89, 90, 91, 93, 94 (cookies and pasta), 95 (beans and ice cream), 96, 98, 102, 103, 123 (Splenda), 128, 150, 163, 164, 178, 182, 183

general index

Underscored references indicate sidebars and tables.
Boldfaced references indicate photographs.

A

Ab curl and chest press, 24, **24**
Abdominal exercises
   ball push-up, 14, **14**
   bicycle, 14, **14**
   crossover, 15, **15**
   hip raise, 17, **17**
   hover, 13, **13**
   instant belly toner, <u>17</u>
   leg raise, 16, **16**
   roll-like-a-ball, 13, **13**
   seated body lift, 17, **17**
   side plank, 15, **15**
   tilt, 16, **16**
Abdominal muscles
   appearance and, <u>16</u>
   exercises for, 12–19, **13–19**, 37, **37**
   importance of strength in, <u>14</u>
   posture and, <u>15</u>
Advanced step-up, 31, **31**
Aerobic exercise, 52–63. *See also* Aerobic workouts
   benefits of, 41
   equipment, <u>60–61</u>
Aerobic workouts. *See also* Aerobic exercise
   bicycling, 53
   classes and videotapes, 52
   elliptical training, 53–54
   hiking, 54
   jogging, 56
   jumping rope, 56–57
   snowshoeing, 57
   stairclimbing machines, 58–59
   stationary cycling, 58
   stepping machines, 58–59
   swimming, 59–62
   tennis, 62
   treadmill running, 56
   walking, 63
Afterburn, 5
Age spot faders, 174
Aging
   effects of diet on, <u>97</u>
   gracefully, <u>78</u>
   muscle loss and, <u>29</u>
Anger, exercise and, 166
Attitudes that interfere with fitness, <u>158</u>

B

Back. *See also* Spine
   exercises for
      back fly, 33, **33**
      one-arm row, 35, **35**
      push-up, 34, **34**
   strengthening, <u>18</u>
   stretches for, 70–71, **71**
Back extension, 21, **21**
Back fly, 33, **33**
Ball crunch, 37, **37**
Ballet exercises, 18–19, **18–19**
   butterfly & heel beat, 18, **18**
   dead bug, 19, **19**
   mermaid, 19, **19**
   pelvic stabilizer, 19, **19**

Ball push-up, 14, **14**
Balls, 163, **163**
Baseball, injury prevention and, 55
Basketball, injury prevention and, 55
Biceps, exercises for
    biceps curl, 23, **23**, 36, **36**
Bicycle (abdominal exercise), 14, **14**
Bicycling, 53
    injury prevention and, 55
Biofoam rollers, 164, **164**
Blood sugar, exercise and, 41
Bone health
    exercise and, 41
    osteoporosis prevention, 35
    strength training and, 5
Butterfly & heel beat, 18, **18**
Butterfly stretch, 30, **30**

C
Calf raise, 11, **11**
Calorie(s)
    burn counts, 41
        aerobic classes and videotapes, 52
        bicycling, 53
        calculating daily requirement,
            105
        elliptical training, 53
        hiking, 54
        jogging, 56
        jumping rope, 56
        snowshoeing, 57
        stairclimbing machines, 58
        stationary cycling, 58
        stepping machines, 58
        swimming, 59
        tennis, 62
        treadmill running, 56
        walking, 63
Calves, stretches for, 68, **68**
Cancer protection, exercise and, 41

Carbohydrate(s), 87–89
    blockers, 87
    in seafood, 98
    weight gain and, 89
    whole grain guide, 88
Cardiovascular exercise. *See also* Cardiovascular
        workouts
    benefits of, 41, 42
    cellulite reduction and, 27
Cardiovascular workouts. *See also*
        Cardiovascular exercise
    beginnings and endings, 46
    personalizing, 47–50
    steps to success, 42–43
Cat pose, 81, **81**
Cellulite reduction, 26–31
    dieting and, 27
    exercises for
        advanced step-up, 31, **31**
        dumbbell squat, 28, **28**
        glute buster, 30
        inner thigh press, 30, **30**
        lunge, 29, **29**
        lying hamstring stretch, 28, **28**
        scissors press, 31, **31**
        standing quadriceps stretch, 29, **29**
Chair dip, 22, **22**
Chest muscles
    exercises for
        chest press, 33, **33**
        push-up, 34, **34**
    stretches for, 70, **70**
Chest fly, 10, **10**
Chest press, 33, **33**
Child's pose, 83, **83**
Cleansers for skin care, 172
Clothing for workouts, 180–83
    bras, 182
    hats, 182
    shirts, 182
    shoes, 183, **183**

shorts, 182
skorts, 181, **181**
socks, 181–83, **182**
Cobra pose, 82, **82**
Cow pose, 82, **82**
Crunch, 22, **22**
Crunchless fab-ab plan, 12–19, **12–19**
Curl and press, 25, **25**

D

Dead bug, 19, **19**
Depression, exercise and, 166
"De-slump" stretch, 75, **75**
Desserts, stocking up, 150
Diagonal curl-up, 11, **11**
Dieting. *See also* Low-carbohydrate eating;
    Weight loss plan
  cellulite and, 27
  tips, 150
Downward dog pose, 80, **80**
Dumbbell squat, 28, **28**

E

Eggs, 98
Elliptical training, 53–54
Emotions, exercise and, 165–67
Equipment
  aerobic exercise, 60–61
  balls, 163, **163**
  biofoam rollers, 164, **164**
  elliptical trainer, 53
  foot massage guide, 163, **163**
  heart rate monitors, 44–45
  jumping rope, 163, **163**
  music packs, 163, **163**
  orthotics, 164, **164**
  pedometer, 164, **164**
  sunscreen, 164, **164**
  tubing, 164, **164**

  water packs, 163, **163**
  wrist water bottles, 182
Exercise(s)
  abdominal muscles, 12–19, **13–19**
  aerobic, 52–63
  back, 18
  ballet, 18–19, **18–19**
  cellulite reduction, 27–31
  gadgets (*see* Equipment)
  motivations for, 154–59, 160–61
  strength training, 6–11, **6–11**
  stretching
    calves, 68, **68**
    chest, 70, **70**
    hamstrings, 68, **68**
    hip flexors, 69, **69**
    hips, 71, **71**
    lower back, 69, **69**
    quadriceps, 69, **69**
    shoulders, 70, **70**
    sides, 69, **69**
    triceps, 69, **69**
    upper back, 70–71, **70–71**
    upper body, 33–37, **33–37**
Eyes, puffy, care for, 175

F

Fat in diet, 100–103
Feet
  massage guide, 163, **163**
  orthotics, 164, **164**
  shoes, 183, **183**
Fiber in diet, importance of, 87–88
Fish, 98
Flexibility training. *See also* Stretching
  for cellulite reduction, 28

G

Glute buster, 30
Glycemic index of foods, 94–95

Golf, injury prevention and, 55
"Goodbye achy back" stretch, 78, **78**

H

Hair care, 176–79
  cuts, 177–79
  dyes, 179
  moisturizers, 178
  thinning, 177
Hamstring, stretches for, 68, **68**
Hamstring curl, 8, **8**
Happiness, exercise and, 167
Heart rate, 44–45
  monitors, 44–45
Hiking, 54
Hip flexors, stretches for, 69, **69**
Hip raise, 17, **17**
Hips, stretches for, 71, **71**
Hover, 13, **13**
Hunchback remover stretch, 76, **76**

I

Injury prevention, 55
In-line skating, injury prevention and, 55
Inner thigh press, 30, **30**

J

Jogging, 56
  injury prevention and, 55
Joint pain, exercise adjustments for, 9
Jumping rope, 56–57
  ropes for, 163, **163**

L

Lateral raise, 23, **23**
Leg raise, 16, **16**
Lifestyle, skin care and, 171–72
Low-carbohydrate eating, 86–95
  food pyramid, 105
  portion sizes, 90–91

  salads, 89
  7-day meal plan, 111–17
  staples to stock, 120–21
  whole grain guide, 88
Lower-back stretches, 69, **69**
Lunge, 7, **7**, 29, **29**
Lying figure-four stretch, 31, **31**
Lying glute stretch, 31, **31**
Lying hamstring stretch, 28, **28**
Lying rotation pose, 83, **83**

M

Masks for skin care, 174–75
Meal plans, 111–17
Meat, choosing, 97
Menus, 111–17
Mermaid, 19, **19**
Metabolism
  exercise and, 41
  weight control and, 5
Military press, 36, **36**
Moisturizers
  hair, 178
  skin, 173
Moods, exercise and, 165–67
Muscle loss, 29
Music packs, 163, **163**

N

Nuts, 98–99
  calories and carbohydrates in, 99

O

One-arm row, 35, **35**
One-leg lunge, 21, **21**
Orthotics, 164, **164**
Osteoporosis prevention, 35

P

Pedometer, 164, **164**
Peels for skin care, 174–75

Pelvic stabilizer, 19, **19**
Pelvic tilt, 16, **16**
Plié, 6, **6**
Portion sizes, 90–91
Posture
  importance of good, 15
  sitting, 23
Poultry, choosing, 87–98
Protein in diet, 96–99
Pullover, 9, **9**
Push-up, 21, **21**, 34, **34**

Q
Quadriceps, stretches for, 69, **69**

R
Rectus abdominis muscle, 16
Resistance machines, 5
Reverse curl, 10, **10**
Roll-like-a-ball, 13, **13**
Running, injury prevention and,
    55

S
Salads, low-carbohydrate, 89
Scissors press, 31, **31**
Seafood, carbohydrates in, 98
Seated body lift, 17, **17**
Seated leg lift, 8, **8**
Seated row, 23, **23**
Shoes for workouts, 183, **183**
Shoulders
  exercises for
    military press, 36, **36**
  stretches for, 70, **70**
Side plank, 15, **15**
Sides, stretches for, 69, **69**
Sitting, posture for, 23

Skin care, 170–75
  products
    age spot faders, 174
    cleansers, 172
    masks and peels, 174–75
    milk-based, 171
    moisturizers, 173
    sunscreen, 164, **164**, 171–72
    vitamin lotions, 173
    wrinkle erasers, 173–74
  regimen, 172–75
Skorts, 181, **181**
Smoking, 172
Snacks
  calories and fats in, 102–3
  low-carbohydrate, 107
Snowshoeing, 57
Soccer, injury prevention and, 55
Socks for workouts, 181–83, **182**
Softball, injury prevention and, 55
Spine, upper body exercises and, 35
Splenda, 123
Squat and side lift, 24, **24**
Stairclimbing
  benefits of, 59
  machines, 58–59
Standing crossover, 15, **15**
Standing quadriceps stretch, 29, **29**
"Stand up straight" stretch, 77, **77**
Stationary cycling, 58
Stepping machines, 58–59
Step and squeeze, 25, **25**
Stess, exercise and, 166
Stevia, 123
Strength training, 4–11. *See also* Strength
    training exercises
  cellulite reduction and, 28
  depression and, 159
  metabolism and, 5
  routine, 6–11, **6–11**
  stretching and, 34

Strength training exercises
  calf raise, 11, **11**
  chest fly, 10, **10**
  diagonal curl-up, 11, **11**
  hamstring curl, 8, **8**
  joint pain adjustments, <u>9</u>
  lunge, 7, **7**
  plié, 6, **6**
  pullover, 9, **9**
  reverse curl, 10, **10**
  seated leg lift, 8, **8**
  triceps kickback, 10, **10**
Stress
  matching stretches to, <u>76</u>
  reduction
    stretching and, 10, <u>77</u>
    yoga and, 79, <u>82</u>
Stretches. *See also* Stretching
  bending chest, <u>34</u>
  butterfly, 30, **30**
  calves, 68, **68**
  cellulite reduction, 30–31,
    30–31
  chest, 70, **70**
  "de-slump," 75, **75**
  "goodbye achy back," 78, **78**
  hamstrings, 68, **68**
  hip flexors, 69, **69**
  hips, 71, **71**
  hunchback remover, 76, **76**
  lower back, 69, **69**
  lying figure-four, 31, **31**
  lying glute stretch, 31, **31**
  quadriceps, 69, **69**
  shoulder(s), <u>34</u>, 70, **70**
  "stand up straight," 77, **77**
  sides, 69, **69**
  triceps, 69, **69**
  upper back, <u>34</u>, 70–71, **70–71**
  "walk with confidence," 75, **75**

Stretching. *See also* Stretches
  benefits of, 67
  customizing routine, <u>76</u>
  how to, <u>72–73</u>
  strength training and, <u>34</u>
  stress relief with, 74–78
Sugar, substitutes for, <u>123</u>
Sunscreen, 164, **164**, 171–72
Swimming, 59–62

T

Tea bags for puffy eyes, 175
10-minute total-body workout, 20–25, **21–25**
Tennis, 62
  injury prevention and, <u>55</u>
Tension, effects of, <u>67</u>
Treadmill running, 56
Triceps
  exercises for
    chest press, 33, **33**
    push-up, 34, **34**
    triceps extension, 37, **37**
  stretches for, 69, **69**
Triceps extension, 22, **22**, 37, **37**
Triceps kickback, 10, **10**
Tubing, 164, **164**

U

Underwear for workouts, 180
Upper back
  exercises for
    back fly, 33, **33**
  stretches for, 70–71, **70–71**
Upper-body exercises, 33–37, **33–37**
  back fly, 33, **33**
  ball crunch, 37, **37**
  biceps curl, 36, **36**
  chest press, 33, **33**

military press, 36, **36**
one-arm row, 35, **35**
push-up, 34, **34**
triceps extension, 37, **37**

V

Vitamin lotions for skin, <u>173</u>
Volleyball, injury prevention and, <u>55</u>

W

"Walk with confidence" stretch, 75, **75**
Walking, 63
Warrior pose, 80, **80**
Water, skin care and, 171
Water aerobics, <u>52</u>
Water packs, 163, **163**
Weight gain, carbohydrates and, 89
Weight lifting. *See* Strength training
Weight loss plan
    carbohydrates in, 106–7
    customizing, 104–7
    FAQs, 118–19
    fats in, 107
    servings of food, <u>106</u>
    7-day meal plan, <u>111–17</u>
    substitutions, <u>107</u>
Workouts
    aerobic
        bicycling, 53
        classes and videotapes, 52
        elliptical training, 53–54
        hiking, 54
        jogging, 56
        jumping rope, 56–57
        showshoeing, 57
        stairclimbing machines, 58–59
        stationary cycling, 58
        stepping machines, 58–59

swimming, 59–62
        tennis, 62
        treadmill running, 56
        walking, 63
    cardiovascular
        beginnings and endings, <u>46</u>
        personalizing, 47–50
        steps to success, 42–46
    clothing for, 180–83
    total body
        ab curl and chest press, 24, **24**
        back extension, 21, **21**
        biceps curl, 23, **23**
        chair dip, 22, **22**
        combination moves, 24–25, **24–25**
        crunch, 22, **22**
        curl and press, 25, **25**
        lateral raise, 23, **23**
        one-leg lunge, 21, **21**
        push-up, 21, **21**
        seated row, 23, **23**
        squat and side lift, 24, **24**
        step and squeeze, 25, **25**
        triceps extension, 22, **22**
    10-minute total-body workout, 20-25, **21–25**
Wrinkle erasers, 173–74

Y

Yoga, 79–83
    benefits of, 79
    do's and don'ts, <u>81</u>
    poses
        cat, 81, **81**
        child's pose, 83, **83**
        cobra, 82, **82**
        cow, 82, **82**
        downward dog, 80, **80**
        lying rotation, 83, **83**
        warrior, 80, **80**

recipe index

Boldface references indicate photographs.

A

Almonds
Raspberry-Almond Tart, 151, **151**
Apples
Baked Apples, 126, **126**
Turkey Sandwich with Swiss Cheese and
Apple, 130, **130**

B

Bacon
Open-Face Bacon-Mushroom Melt, 131,
131
Bananas
Cantauloupe Sorbet, 145, **145**
Whole Grain Crepes with Banana and
Kiwifruit, 125, **125**
Beef
Filet Mignon with Tomatoes and Rosemary,
140, **140**
Meat Loaf with Walnuts, 142, **142**
Roast Beef Sandwich with
Mustard-Horseradish Mayonnaise, 128,
128
Smothered Pot Roast, 141, **141**
Biscotti
Orange-Walnut Biscotti, 146, **146**
Blueberries
Peach Soufflé with Blueberries, 153,
153

Breakfast, 122–27
Baked Apples, 126, **126**
Cherry Cream of Rye Cereal, 123,
123
Fried Eggs with Vinegar, 122, **122**
Pecan Muffins, 124, **124**
Puffy Frittata with Ham and Green Pepper,
127, **127**
Whole Grain Crepes with Banana and
Kiwifruit, 125, **125**
Broccoli
Creamy Broccoli Soup with Chicken, 133,
133
Stir-Fried Chicken and Broccoli, 136,
136

C

Cabbage
Pork Chops Baked with Cabbage and Cream,
135, **135**
Two-Cheese Pita Melt, 130
Cakes
Chocolate Hazelnut Flourless Cake, 152,
152
Gingerbread Cake with Peach Whipped
Cream, 148, **148**
Strawberry Cream Cake, 149, **149**
Cantaloupe
Cantaloupe Sorbet, 145, **145**

Cereal
  Cherry Cream of Rye Cereal, 123,
    123
Cheese
  Chicken Parmesan, 143, **143**
  Open-Face Bacon-Mushroom Melt, 131,
    131
  Pesto Chicken Sandwich with Roasted
    Peppers, 132, **132**
  Turkey Cutlets with Ham and Provolone, 144,
    144
  Turkey Sandwich with Swiss Cheese and
    Apple, 130, **130**
  Two-Cheese Pita Melt, 130
Cherries
  Cherry Cream of Rye Cereal, 123,
    123
Chicken
  Chicken Parmesan, 143, **143**
  Creamy Broccoli Soup with Chicken, 133,
    133
  Chicken Sandwich with Roasted Peppers, 132,
    132
  Stir-Fried Chicken and Broccoli, 136,
    136
Chocolate
  Chocolate Hazelnut Flourless Cake, 152,
    152
  Double Chocolate Pudding, 150, **150**
Cod
  Breaded Baked Cod with Tartar Sauce, 137,
    137
Cookies
  Orange-Walnut Biscotti, 146, **146**
  Peanut Butter Cookies, 147, **147**
Crepes
  Whole Grain Crepes with Banana and
    Kiwifruit, 125, **125**

D
Desserts, 145–53
  Cantaloupe Sorbet, 145, **145**
  Chocolate Hazelnut Flourless Cake, 152,
    152
  Double Chocolate Pudding, 150, **150**
  Gingerbread Cake with Peach Whipped
    Cream, 148, **148**
  Orange-Walnut Biscotti, 146, **146**
  Peach Soufflé with Blueberries, 153,
    153
  Peanut Butter Cookies, 147, **147**
  Raspberry-Almond Tart, 151, **151**
  Strawberry Cream Cake, 149, **149**
Dinner, 134-44
  Breaded Baked Cod with Tartar Sauce, 137,
    137
  Chicken Parmesan, 143, **143**
  Filet Mignon with Tomatoes and Rosemary,
    140, **140**
  Meat Loaf with Walnuts, 142, **142**
  Mushroom and Kasha Soup, 138, **138**
  Pork Chops Baked with Cabbage and Cream,
    135, **135**
  Scallops in Tarragon Cream, 139, **139**
  Smothered Pot Roast, 141, **141**
  Spanish Style-Green Beans, 134, **134**
  Stir-Fried Chicken and Broccoli, 136,
    136
  Turkey Cutlets with Ham and Provolone, 144,
    144

E
Eggs
  Fried Eggs with Vinegar, 122, **122**
  Puffy Frittata with Ham and Green Pepper,
    127, **127**

Eggs *(cont.)*
Sausage, Egg, and Vegetable Casserole, 129, **129**

F
Fish
Breaded Baked Cod with Tartar Sauce, 137, **137**

G
Green beans
Spanish Style-Green Beans, 134, **134**

H
Ham
Puffy Frittata with Ham and Green Pepper, 127, **127**
Turkey Cutlets with Ham and Provolone, 144, **144**
Hazelnuts
Chocolate Hazelnut Flourless Cake, 152, **152**
Horseradish
Roast Beef Sandwich with Mustard-Horseradish Mayonnaise, 128, **128**

K
Kasha
Mushroom and Kasha Soup, 138, **138**
Kiwifruit
Whole Grain Crepes with Banana and Kiwifruit, 125, **125**

L
Lunch, 128–33
Creamy Broccoli Soup with Chicken, 133, **133**
Open-Face Bacon-Mushroom Melt, 131, **131**
Pesto Chicken Sandwich with Roasted Peppers, 132, **132**
Roast Beef Sandwich with Mustard-Horseradish Mayonnaise, 128, **128**
Sausage, Egg, and Vegetable Casserole, 129, **129**
Turkey Sandwich with Swiss Cheese and Apple, 130, **130**
Two-Cheese Pita Melt, 130

M
Muffins
Pecan Muffins, 124, **124**
Mushrooms
Mushroom and Kasha Soup, 138, **138**
Open-Face Bacon-Mushroom Melt, 131, **131**
Mustard
Roast Beef Sandwich with Mustard-Horseradish Mayonnaise, 128, **128**

N
Nuts
Chocolate Hazelnut Flourless Cake, 152, **152**
Meat Loaf with Walnuts, 142, **142**
Orange-Walnut Biscotti, 146, **146**

Pecan Muffins, 124, **124**
Raspberry-Almond Tart, 151, **151**

O
Oranges
Orange-Walnut Biscotti, 146, **146**

P
Peaches
Gingerbread Cake with Peach Whipped
Cream, 148, **148**
Peach Soufflé with Blueberries, 153,
153
Peanut butter
Peanut Butter Cookies, 147, **147**
Pecans
Pecan Muffins, 124, **124**
Peppers, bell
Puffy Frittata with Ham and Green Pepper,
127, **127**
Peppers, roasted
Pesto Chicken Sandwich with Roasted
Peppers, 132, **132**
Pesto
Pesto Chicken Sandwich with Roasted
Peppers, 132, **132**
Pork
Pork Chops Baked with Cabbage and Cream,
135, **135**
Pudding
Double Chocolate Pudding, 150, **150**

R
Raspberries
Raspberry-Almond Tart, 151, **151**

Rosemary
Filet Mignon with Tomatoes and Rosemary,
140, **140**
Rye
Cherry Cream of Rye Cereal, 123, **123**

S
Sandwiches
Open-Face Bacon-Mushroom Melt, 131,
131
Pesto Chicken Sandwich with Roasted
Peppers, 132, **132**
Roast Beef Sandwich with
Mustard-Horseradish Mayonnaise, 128,
128
Turkey Sandwich with Swiss Cheese and
Apple, 130, **130**
Two-Cheese Pita Melt, 130
Sausages
Sausage, Egg, and Vegetable Casserole, 129,
129
Scallops
Scallops in Tarragon Cream, 139, **139**
Sorbet
Cantaloupe Sorbet, 145, **145**
Soups
Creamy Broccoli Soup with Chicken, 133,
133
Mushroom and Kasha Soup, 138, **138**
Strawberries
Strawberry Cream Cake, 149,
149

T
Tarragon
Scallops in Tarragon Cream, 139, **139**

Tart
    Raspberry-Almond Tart, 151, **151**
Tomatoes
    Chicken Parmesan, 143, **143**
    Filet Mignon with Tomatoes and Rosemary,
       140, **140**
Tortillas
    Pesto Chicken Sandwich with Roasted
       Peppers, 132, **132**
Turkey
    Turkey Cutlets with Ham and Provolone, 144,
       144
    Sandwich with Swiss Cheese and Apple, 130,
       130

V
Vegetables. *See also specific kinds*
    Sausage, Egg, and Vegetable Casserole, 129,
       129
Vinegar
    Fried Eggs with Vinegar, 122, **122**

W
Walnuts
    Meat Loaf with Walnuts, 142,
       142
    Orange-Walnut Biscotti, 146,
       146